MW01119589

Criminal Justice
Recent Scholarship

Edited by
Nicholas P. Lovrich

A Series from LFB Scholarly

TASERs and Arrest-Related Deaths

Howard E. Williams

LFB Scholarly Publishing LLC
El Paso 2015

Copyright © 2015 by LFB Scholarly Publishing LLC

Library of Congress Cataloging-in-Publication Data

Library of Congress Cataloging-in-Publication Data

Williams, Howard E., author.
 TASERs and arrest-related deaths / Howard E. Williams.
   p. ; cm.
 Includes bibliographical references and index.
 ISBN 978-1-59332-788-0 (hardcover : alk. paper)
 I. Title.
 [DNLM: 1. Autopsy--methods--United States. 2. Forensic
Pathology--methods--United States. 3. Conducted Energy Weapon
Injuries--mortality--United States. 4. Death, Sudden--etiology--United
States. 5. Police--United States. W 825]
 RB57
 RA1063.4--dc23
                          2014039078

ISBN 978-1-59332-788-0

Manufactured in the United States of America.

Table of Contents

List of Tables vi

List of Figures vii

List of Acronyms and Abbreviations ix

Acknowledgements xiii

Preface xv

Chapter 1: Arrest-Related Sudden Death and High-Risk Group
Theory 1

Chapter 2: What We Know About Arrest-Related Sudden Death 19

Chapter 3: What We Know About TASER Technology 39

Chapter 4: Testing High-Risk Group Theory 87

Chapter 5: Research Findings 105

Chapter 6: Implications and Conclusions 137

Appendix A: Search Terms 157

Appendix B: Coding Instrument 159

Appendix C: Coding Instrument Instructions 163

Appendix D: STATA Regression Model Tables 169

Glossary 173

References 181

Cases Cited 207

Index 209

List of Tables

Table 1. Ratio of ECD Arrest-Related Sudden Deaths by Year.........107

Table 2. Logistic Regression Analysis of Attribute Data...................109

Table 3. Age Data for Arrest-Related Sudden Deaths 111

Table 4. χ^2 Contingency Table for Sex 112

Table 5. χ^2 Contingency Table for Race/Ethnicity............................113

Table 6. χ^2 Contingency Table for Cardiovascular Disease...............114

Table 7. χ^2 Contingency Table for Drugs Present..............................116

Table 8. χ^2 Contingency Table for Amphetamines Present...............117

Table 9. χ^2 Contingency Table for Cocaine Present..........................118

Table 10. χ^2 Contingency Table for Marijuana Present 119

Table 11. χ^2 Contingency Table for Opiates Present..........................119

Table 12. χ^2 Contingency Table for PCP Present...............................120

Table 13. χ^2 Contingency Table for History of Drug Abuse..............121

Table 14. χ^2 Contingency Table for Excited Delirium.......................122

Table 15. χ^2 Contingency Table for Alcohol Present.........................123

Table 16. χ^2 Contingency Table for Chronic Alcohol Abuse.............124

Table 17. χ^2 Contingency Table for Mental Illness............................126

Table 18. χ^2 Contingency Table for Psychotropic Medications.........127

Table 19. csQCA Case Configurations by Cell Frequency..............129

Table 20. Summary of Findings...136

List of Figures

Figure 1. Total Arrest-Related Sudden Deaths by Year...................... 106
Figure 2. Non-ECD versus ECD-Proximate Arrest-Related
      Sudden Deaths by Year... 106

List of Acronyms and Abbreviations

AED	Automatic external defibrillator
AH	History of amphetamine use
AP	Amphetamine present
BJS	Bureau of Justice Statistics
BPM	Beats per minute
C	Centigrade
CH	History of cocaine use
CI	Confidence interval
cm	Centimeter
CO_2	Carbon dioxide
Con	Consistency
CONS	Constant
CP	Cocaine present
csQCA	Crisp set Qualitative Comparative Analysis
CT	Computed tomography
CVD	Cardiovascular disease
d	Cohen's d
DAP	Drugs present
DCRP	Deaths in Custody Reporting Program
dL	Deciliter
DOMILL	Defence Scientific Advisory Sub-Committee on Less-Lethal Weapons
ECD	Electronic control device
ETOH	Alcohol present
ExDS	Excited delirium syndrome
F	Fahrenheit
FBI	Federal Bureau of Investigation

Freq	Frequency
fsQCA	Fuzzy set Qualitative Comparative Analysis
HCAA	History of chronic alcohol abuse
HDA	History of drug abuse
HPA	Hypothalamus-pituitary-adrenal
ICD	Implantable cardioverter-defibrillator
j	Joule
K	Kappa
kg	Kilograms
L	Liter
LH	History of LSD use
LP	LSD present
LR	Likelihood ratio
m	Minute
mA	Milliamp
MDMA	3,4-methylenedioxy-4- methamphetamine
mg	Milligram
MH	History of marijuana use
MI	Myocardial infarction
mL	Milliliter
mm	Millimeter
MNIL	Mental illness plus psychotropic medications
MP	Marijuana present
ms	Millisecond
MT	Mental illness
mvQCA	Multiple value Qualitative Comparative Analysis
μC	Microcoulomb
μs	Microsecond
ng	Nanogram
NVDRS	National Violent Death Reporting System
O_2	Oxygen
OC	Oleoresin capsicum
OH	History of opiates use
OP	Opiates present
O.R.	Odds ratio
pCO_2	Partial pressure of carbon dioxide
PEA	Pulseless electrical activity
PERF	Police Executive Research Forum
PH	History of PCP use

PMED	Psychotropic medications
pO_2	Partial pressure of oxygen
PP	PCP present
PPS	Pulses per second
QCA	Qualitative Comparative Analysis
r	Effect size correlation
RR	Respiration rate
SAM	Sympathetic-adrenal-medulla
TdP	Torsade de pointes
UCR	Uniform Crime Reports
V	Volt
VF	Ventricular fibrillation
VT	Ventricular tachycardia
WISQRS	Web-Based Injury Statistics Query and Reporting System
WODER	Wide-Ranging Online Data for Epidemiologic Research
χ^2	Chi-square

Acknowledgements

I wish, first, to thank Joycelyn Pollock, J. Pete Blair, Brian Withrow, and Michael D. White for their assistance in designing and developing this research. I sincerely appreciate their diligence, their thoroughness, their candor, and their patience as I conceptualized and then conducted the study reported here. Additionally, Kelly Williams and Nick Icossipentarhos volunteered many hours of their valuable time to code reports.

Most importantly, I thank my wife, Kelly, for thirty years of love and support. She sacrifices much to accommodate my careers in law enforcement and academics. I could not succeed in either endeavor without her, and I am forever indebted to her.

Preface

TASER electronic control devices (ECDs), manufactured by TASER International, Inc. in Scottsdale, Arizona, have become a popular tool for law enforcement. TASER International has sold more than 710,000 devices to 16,880 agencies in 107 countries. Although other manufacturers produce comparable types of electro-shock weapons, TASER products are the most commonly used in the United States and worldwide.

Unfortunately, more than 900 people worldwide have died unexpectedly following law enforcement officers' uses of TASER ECDs. Currently, there is no research definitively establishing a causal relationship between the use of an ECD and the death of a person exposed to it. However, some recent studies suggest that application of TASER technology is responsible for sudden unexpected deaths. The ever increasing number of deaths following application of TASER ECDs and the growing number of cases wherein a coroner or medical examiner attribute the use of an ECD as a cause of death or as a significant contributing factor to the death raise legitimate concerns about the safety threshold of the devices.

Researchers have proposed and tested many theories of why people die following the application of ECDs, including direct electro-stimulation of cardiac muscle, interference with breathing, and metabolic changes resulting in acidosis. Thus far, human model experiments have produced no evidence to support these theories. Another theory, which has recently appeared in the literature, has received no empirical testing—the theory of high-risk groups. High-risk group theory postulates that elderly people, young children, people with pre-existing cardiovascular disease, people with pacemakers and implantable cardioverter-defibrillators, people under the influence of drugs (amphetamines, cocaine, lysergic acid diethylamide, marijuana, opiates, and/or phencyclidine) or with a history of drug abuse, people intoxicated from alcohol or with a history of chronic alcohol abuse, people under extreme psychological distress or who exhibit signs of excited delirium, people who are mentally ill or taking psychotropic medications, people subjected to repeated or multiple applications, and pregnant women are at a heightened risk of serious injury or death following application of a TASER ECD.

What the current literature fails to consider is that the same physiological attributes that are presumed to render members of high-risk groups more vulnerable to serious injury or death following application of a TASER ECD might render these same people more vulnerable to serious injury or death regardless of the tactics or weapons that officers use to subdue them. If that hypothesis is correct, the use of TASER ECDs on people in high-risk groups might be irrelevant to arrest-related sudden deaths.

The potential for fatal adverse effects on high-risk groups when using other less lethal tactics and methods versus the potential for fatal adverse effects on high-risk groups following the use of a TASER ECD is currently unknown. Thus far, research has not directly addressed that question. By examining autopsy and toxicology reports of the deceased and comparing differences in the physiological attributes of arrest-related sudden deaths, one can then estimate whether a difference exists in high-risk group attributes between deaths proximate to the use of a TASER ECD and deaths not involving the use of an ECD.

This study examines physiological attributes in arrest-related sudden deaths. An arrest-related sudden death is a death that occurs following a collapse within 24 hours after the initial arrest or detention. The death must be unexpected, must not be the result of trauma or injury that a layperson could readily discern needs medical attention, and must follow a sudden change in clinical condition or the beginning of symptoms from which the deceased does not recover. It does not include ovious trauma deaths, police shootings, or suicides.

This work was a retrospective open source research study of publicly available autopsy and toxicology reports designed to compare the physiological attributes of high-risk group theory to two groups of arrest-related sudden deaths, TASER ECD-proximate deaths and non-ECD deaths. A non-proportional stratified random sample of 300 publicly available reports was obtained for study and coded for physiological attributes of high-risk groups. Descriptive and inferential quantitative statistics, specifically Student's *t*-test, Pearson's chi-square, and bivariate logistic regression (logit) were used to analyze the data and compare attributes for any significant differences observed. Additionally, crisp set Qualitative Comparative Analysis (csQCA) was used to examine whether any configuration of causal conditions described a unique path to arrest-related sudden death following application of a TASER ECD.

The study included data on 1,060 arrest-related sudden deaths that occurred in the United States between January 1, 2006 and December 31, 2011. The results indicate that the physiological attributes of TASER-proximate deaths look much like the attributes in non-ECD deaths. The one notable exception was the statistically significant difference in deaths involving excited delirium syndrome.

CHAPTER 1

Arrest-Related Sudden Death and High-Risk Group Theory

TASER® electronic control devices, manufactured by TASER International, Inc. in Scottsdale, Arizona, have become a popular tool for law enforcement since Jack Cover patented and sold the first device in 1974 (Smith, 2006).[1] Almost 40 years of technological development have produced several generations of TASER products. Earlier generation devices included the TF-76™, the TASERTRON™, the AIR TASER 34000™, the M18™, the ADVANCED TASER® M26™, and, briefly, the XREP™. Only the later generation models, the X26™, the X2™, the X3™, and the C2™, were in production at the end of 2012.[2] By the end of that year, TASER International had sold more than 710,000 devices to 16,880 law enforcement and corrections agencies in 107 countries (Kukowski, 2012). Terrill, Paoline, and Ingram (2012), in a national survey of police agencies, found that approximately 80 percent of the 662 responding agencies in the United States reported that they were using electronic control devices.

Although other manufacturers produce comparable types of electro-shock weapons, TASER products are the most commonly used in the United States and worldwide, and TASER technology has undergone the most extensive domestic and international scientific testing

---

[1] TASER® and ADVANCED TASER® are trademarks of TASER International, Inc., registered in the United States. All rights reserved.
[2] TF-76™, TASERTRON™, AIR TASER 34000™, M18™, M26™, XREP™, X26™, X2™, X3™, and C2™ are trademarks of TASER International, Inc.

related to its safety, efficacy, and risk utility (Peters, 2006). Consequently, because other manufacturers use different electro-shock technologies, because so few deaths have followed the application of other manufacturers' products, and because there is so little research on the effects of other electronic control technologies, this study examines only the effects of TASER-brand name devices. Any death involving another brand name device will not be a death related to a TASER electronic control device, although, depending on the circumstances, it might be an arrest-related sudden death.

Researchers and authors have used many terms to describe TASER products, including neuromuscular incapacitating devices, conducted energy weapons, conductive electrical devices, electronic control weapons, and electronic control devices. For the sake of simplicity, the term *electronic control device* and its acronym ECD are used here.

The TASER X26, the X2, and the X3 are the models that law enforcement agencies now use almost exclusively. These devices deliver a five-second electrical charge of 19 pulses per second (PPS), each pulse lasting approximately 100 microseconds (μs). The average peak loaded voltage over the duration of the main phase is 1200 volts (V), with an average over the full phase of about 350 V. The electrical current averages 2.1 milliamps (mA) and delivers about 0.07 joules (J) of energy into the load. The device also generates an open-circuit voltage of up to 50,000 V to arc through air or through thick clothing, but the ECD does not deliver 50,000 V to the body (Kroll, 2009; Kunz, Zinka, Fieseler, Graw, and Peschel, 2012).

TASER ECDs operate in three ways: probe mode, drive-stun mode, and a hybrid mode. The probe mode uses compressed nitrogen to propel two electrodes toward a target. A pseudo-monophasic waveform electrical signal transmits through connected wires to where the probes make contact with the body or with clothing. A pseudo-monophasic pulse is a biphasic pulse in which the second phase duration is much greater than the first. Optimal results of the probe mode include immediate loss of neuromuscular control and loss of the ability to coordinate muscular actions for the five-second duration of the electric impulse (Panescu, Kroll, and Stratbucker, 2009).

The drive-stun mode results from pressing the electrodes of the ECD directly to the skin, thus stimulating A-δ neural fibers to produce a sensation of sharp pain and, thereby, to promote compliance. In the hybrid mode, the electric current passes from a single probe to either or both of the two drive-stun electrodes on the weapon that are in direct contact with the skin (Panescu, et al., 2009). TASER International manufactured its early generations of ECDs from the 1970s through the 1990s. These early devices were essentially pain-compliance tools, but following some product demonstrations wherein test subjects were able to fight through the pain, TASER International developed newer weapons that could interfere with voluntary muscle control (Smith, 2006).

Newer generation TASER ECDs, in production since 1999, employ electro-muscular disruption technology that affects the sensory and motor functions of the somatic nervous system (International Association of Chiefs of Police, 2006). The somatic nervous system is that part of the peripheral nervous system that serves the sense organs and the muscles of the body wall and limbs and that brings about voluntary muscle activity. The peripheral nervous system is that entirety of the nervous system that lies outside the brain and spinal cord. Modern ECDs use electrical stimuli to interfere with peripheral nervous system signals temporarily to impair a subject's ability to control voluntary muscle movement through a phenomenon termed *clonus*—a series of rapid repetitive contractions and relaxations in a muscle during movement (Smith, 2006).

TASER International engineered the 100 μs pulses of the pseudo-monophasic waveform to stimulate A-ἁ motor neurons, the nerves that control skeletal muscle contraction, without stimulating the cardiac muscle (Kroll, 2009). However, Despa, Basati, Zhang, D'Andrea, Reilly, Bodnar, and Lee (2009) theorize that because electrodes in contact with the body activate multiple nerve types in the area of the electrode, the electric pulses might stimulate spinal reflexes. They could not determine whether the impulses influence the central nervous system. Sun and Webster (2007) suggest that stimulation of the spinal cord, and consequently the central nervous system, could occur with probe penetration into the anterior torso.

Studies on the effectiveness of TASER ECDs in field applications have yielded rather mixed results. In a pilot study examining a random selection of 400 deployments, Mesloh, Henych, Hougland, and Thompson (2005) reported TASER ECDs were successful in subduing the suspect without the need for further use of force in 68 percent of incidents. In a subsequent study at a large metropolitan police agency, White and Ready (2007) reported that deployment of TASER ECDs incapacitated 85 percent of suspects, who were then taken into custody without further incident. In studies of deaths following the application of TASER ECDs, however, Williams (2008) found that the ECDs were ineffective in subduing 61.6 percent of 213 people who died subsequent to the application of the ECD. White, Ready, Riggs, Dawes, Hinz, and Ho (2013) found that in 58.4 percent of 392 TASER ECD-proximate deaths the subjects continued to struggle either immediately after the application of the ECD or at some later point in the arrest encounter.

THE LETHALITY DEBATE

Arrest-related sudden deaths occur relatively rarely. In 2008, the latest year for which data are available, police in the United States engaged in approximately 40 million face-to-face encounters with citizens (Eith and Durose, 2011). Subsequent to those encounters, the Bureau of Justice Statistics (BJS), through the Deaths in Custody Reporting Program (DCRP), reported 629 arrest-related deaths (Burch, 2011), which included suicides, officer-involved shootings, and other fatalities that are not arrest-related sudden deaths. Unfortunately, the BJS reports aggregate data in a way that makes disaggregating data on arrest-related sudden deaths impossible. Still, all arrest-related deaths occur in only about 1.57 of every 100,000 police/citizen encounters.

From 2003 through 2009, the Federal Bureau of Investigation (FBI) reports that approximately 97.9 million arrests occurred in the United States. During that same period, the BJS reports 4,813 arrest-related deaths (Burch, 2011). Again, it is impossible to disaggregate data on arrest-related sudden deaths, but all arrest-related deaths occurred in only about 4.92 of every 100,000 arrests. Arrest-related deaths are only a small subset of all deaths, but to put the arrest-related death rates in perspective, the age-adjusted death rate in the United States was 749.6 deaths per 100,000 people in 2009 and 746.2 deaths per 100,000 people in 2010 (Murphy, Xu, and Kochanek, 2012). It is important to note that the FBI's Uniform Crime Reports (UCR) data on arrests do not include detentions for obtaining emergency medical care or detentions for mental health assistance. The DCRP reports that in 3.4 percent of reported deaths from 2003 through 2009 no criminal charges were intended. These deaths occurred during mental health or medical treatment transports (Burch, 2011).

Reports of deaths following the use of ECDs have generated growing public debate over the potentially adverse effects of TASER technology. Public safety concerns arising from this debate affect policy decisions, which, in turn, affect officer and citizen safety. The courts' understanding of potentially adverse effects of the use of TASER ECDs influences legal opinions on issues of liability for wrongful death and culpability for excessive use of force.

The United States Department of Defense defines non-lethal weapons as those explicitly designed and primarily employed to incapacitate personnel while minimizing fatalities and permanent injuries (Maier, Nance, Price, Sherry, Reilly, Klauenberg, and Drummond, 2005). Although TASER ECDs fit within the Department of Defense definition of non-lethal weapons, many law enforcement executives eschew that term in favor of either *less-lethal* or *less-than-lethal* (Police Executive Research Forum and U.S. Department of Justice, 2011). Currently, the generally accepted term is less-lethal, which conveys the sense that, although ECDs are likely to be less injurious than lethal force, a possibility still exists that death or serious injury can occur with the use of those weapons (Sloane and Vilke, 2008).

Currently, there is no research or evidence establishing a causal relationship between the use of an ECD and the death of a person exposed to it (Laub, 2011; Standing Advisory Subcommittee on the Use of Force, 2007; White, et al., 2013). To the contrary, many studies rule out ECDs as the primary cause of deaths following their application (Synyshyn, 2008). Instead, most current research suggests that deaths associated with ECDs are generally attributable to other causes, and that deaths proximate to the application of ECDs are most likely coincidental (Chand and Nash, 2009). However, some recent studies suggest that application of TASER technology is responsible for some sudden unexpected deaths (Lee, Vittinghoff, Whiteman, Park, Lau, and Tseng, 2009; Zipes, 2012).

Fox and Payne-James (2012) modified the Naranjo algorithm, an algorithm popular for testing attribution of pharmaceutical products to serious adverse events, to review 175 deaths proximate to the application of a TASER ECD. They classified 20 cases as probable, and one case as definite. However, they also found that the mode of death in the 20 probable cases was unrelated to the properties of the ECD. Eight fatalities were due to secondary blunt head trauma from falls, and two deaths occurred because of ECD-ignited fires in atmospheres containing flammable vapors. In the ten remaining cases, coroners or medical examiners attributed concomitant cardiovascular disease or drug use as the principal cause of death. From the results of the study, they concluded that some published case fatality rates attributable to ECD exposure were likely exaggerated.

Moreover, several judicial and investigative bodies have dismissed the likelihood that ECDs are responsible for arrest-related deaths. In rendering judgment following a four-day trial to determine whether the use of TASER ECDs was the cause of death for three men in Summit County, Ohio, the trial judge ruled that there was no compelling medical, scientific, or electrical evidence to support a conclusion that TASER ECDs caused those deaths (*TASER International et al. v. Kohler*, 2008). The Ninth Judicial District Court of Appeals upheld that decision, albeit with some changes to the trial court's orders regarding required changes to wording on the death certificates (*TASER International, et al. v. Kohler*, 2009).

In 2008, after experiencing three arrest-related deaths proximate to the use of TASER ECDs in Alleghany County, Pennsylvania over the period 2006 through 2008, the District Attorney convened a working group to study the use of those devices. The working group concluded that, at best, there was insufficient evidence to conclude that careful and judicious use of TASER ECDs caused deaths. The group argued that if TASER ECDs caused more deaths in the course of arrests than other weapons, then historical evidence would have shown a substantial increase in arrest-related deaths after they were introduced; however, no such evidence existed (Harris, 2010).

In 2006, the United States Department of Justice convened a panel of physicians, medical examiners, and specialists in cardiology, emergency medicine, epidemiology, pathology and toxicology to conduct mortality reviews of almost 300 TASER ECD-proximate deaths. The panel reported that there was no conclusive medical evidence to indicate a high risk of serious injury or death from the direct effects of ECD exposure (Laub, 2011; National Institute of Justice, 2008).

However, critics of TASER technology hold that the substantial number of deaths following application of TASER ECDs demonstrate that they are potentially lethal weapons. Those critics note that coroners and medical examiners in several cases identify the use of ECDs as the cause of, or a contributing factor to, the deaths investigated. Amnesty International, a human rights organization and winner of the 1977 Nobel Peace Prize, equates the use of TASER ECDs to the use of deadly force. The organization suggests that law enforcement agencies should restrict the use of ECDs to "situations where officers are faced with an immediate threat of death or serious injury that cannot be contained through less extreme options, in order to avoid the resort to firearms (Amnesty International, 2008a:10)." Although Amnesty International recognizes the need for law enforcement officers to use force in justifiable circumstances, it contends that serious questions remain unanswered concerning safety thresholds of ECDs, and it urges a moratorium on their use pending rigorous independent studies.

Kershaw (2004) first reported on 29 deaths related to the use of TASER ECDs over the period 2001 through 2003. She noted the rising rate of deaths each year—3 in 2001, 10 in 2002, and 16 in 2003. Anglen (2004) reported 44 deaths associated with the use of TASER ECDs in the United States and Canada between September 1999 and March 2004. He noted that coroners or medical examiners listed the use of ECDs as a contributing factor in five of those cases. Amnesty International (2004) published a report that cited 74 deaths following the use of TASER ECDs in the United States and Canada in the period June 2001 through January 2004. In seven of those cases, coroners or medical examiners concluded that either the use of ECDs contributed to the death or they could not rule out their use as a cause or a contributing factor. Barton (2005) reported on 27 TASER ECD-proximate deaths in Florida occurring between June 2002 and January 2005. Although she noted that cocaine use was involved in 17 of the 27 deaths, she noted that medical examiners had listed the use of an ECD as a contributing factor in three cases, and they could not rule it out in one more.

Two years after his original report, Anglen (2006) published an update that listed 167 deaths in the United States and Canada taking place over the period September 1999 through December 2005. Of those deaths, coroners or medical examiners listed TASER ECDs as the cause of death, as a contributing factor in the death, or were unable to rule out the use of the ECD as a cause of death in 27 cases. At about the same time as the second Anglen report, Amnesty International (2006) published a second report listing 152 deaths in the United States between November 2004 and February 2006 and claimed that medical authorities had listed the use of an ECD as a contributing factor in 26 of those cases.

Williams (2008) published a list of 213 deaths in the United States that occurred from August 1983, the date of the earliest recorded death related to the use of a first generation TASER ECD, through December 2006. Shortly thereafter, Amnesty International (2008b) published a third report listing 334 arrest-related deaths that occurred in the United States between June 2001 and August 2008. Although Amnesty International did not claim that all 334 deaths resulted from the application of ECDs, the report emphasized that in at least 50 cases coroners and medical examiners had listed the use of TASER ECDs as a cause of or as a contributing factor to the death (Amnesty International, 2008a). Most recently, White, et al. (2013) reported incident-level data on 392 arrest-related deaths in the United States involving deployment of an ECD over the period 2001 to 2008.

The ever-increasing number of deaths following application of TASER ECDs and the growing number of cases wherein a coroner or medical examiner has attributed the use of an ECD as the cause of death or as a significant contributing factor to the death raise legitimate concerns about the safety threshold of the devices. Adding to the concerns are reports and studies that conclude that ECDs are capable of causing death.

To address concerns about the arrest-related death of a reportedly healthy young man, Maryland's Attorney General assembled a Task Force on Electronic Weapons to study the effects of TASER ECDs and to recommend best practices for law enforcement. After a year of gathering information and holding public hearings, the task force issued its report urging Maryland's legislature, law enforcement agencies deploying ECDs, and front-line officers to recognize the inherent risks of serious injury and the risks of death from secondary factors such as falls or the stress of being shocked (Higginbotham, Warnken, Snowden, Alves, Boersma, Crawford, Hansel, Hammack, Lopez, Johnson, McKinney, Meekins, Pelton, Ricks, and Warren, 2009).

Lee, et al. (2009) reported survey results on the effects of TASER ECD deployment on rates of in-custody sudden deaths in the absence of lethal force. The study reported data from 50 agencies in California for five years preceding ECD deployment through the five years after ECD deployment. The rate of in-custody sudden death increased 6.4-fold in the first full year after ECD deployment compared with the average rate in the five years before deployment. In subsequent years, however, in-custody death rates decreased to pre-deployment levels. The researchers speculated that liberal use of TASER ECDs in the first year might have contributed to the increased rates, and that later decreases might reflect law enforcement recognition of the potential adverse consequences of ECD application, which led to less frequent use and more limited scope of use.

Following a highly publicized and contentious death involving a TASER ECD in the airport in Vancouver, Canada, the Attorney General of British Columbia ordered an inquest to inquire into and report on the use of TASER ECDs in British Columbia. The commissioner convened 61 days of hearings and received testimony from 91 witnesses. In his report on the inquest, Braidwood (2009) concluded that even in healthy adults TASER ECDs could cause heart arrhythmia, which could lead to ventricular tachycardia (VT), an abnormal heart rhythm that is rapid and regular and that originates from an area of the lower chamber of the heart, and/or ventricular fibrillation (VF), an abnormal and irregular heart rhythm in which there are rapid uncoordinated fluttering contractions of the lower chambers of the heart, a condition which can cause death.

Zipes (2012) reported a case study series in which eight people lost consciousness and suffered cardiac arrhythmia following application of a TASER ECD. Cardiac arrhythmia can be any of a number of problems with the rate or rhythm of the heart that is beating too fast, too slowly, or with an irregular rhythm. Seven of Zipes' cases resulted in the death of the individual, and one individual survived. All of the individuals in question were males who received shocks from an X26 with one or both probes in the chest near or over the heart. On autopsy, pathologists discovered several of the victims had structural heart disease and/or had elevated blood alcohol concentrations. Three toxicology reports were positive for marijuana, and one was positive for medications for a seizure disorder. Zipes concluded that electro-stimulation from the ECD in the presence of structural heart disease and/or alcohol intoxication induced VT or VF. He based his opinion on clinical electrophysiology studies that established that the presence of structural heart disease facilitates electrical induction of VT and VF, as does alcohol.

Although research has not yet established a definitive causal relationship, researchers have proposed and tested many theories of why people might die following the application of ECDs. These theories have included direct electro-stimulation of cardiac muscle, interference with breathing, and metabolic changes resulting in acidosis, an abnormal increase in blood acidity. Thus far, human model experiments have produced no evidence to support these theories (Pasquier, Carron, Vallotton, and Yersin, 2011). Another theory, which has recently appeared in the literature, has not been subjected to empirical testing—namely, *the theory of high-risk groups.*

NAISSANCE OF HIGH-RISK GROUP THEORY

A common theme in recent literature on TASER technology postulates that groups of people who have certain physical and mental attributes are more susceptible to sudden death following the application of ECDs than people who do not possess those attributes. Authors have coined the phrase "high-risk groups" to identify such people. There is no literature formally introducing or defining high-risk group as a unique theory, and no experimental human evidence currently exists to support the theory's assumptions (Bozeman, Winslow, and Hauda, 2009). Nevertheless, despite the lack of a formally proposed theory or empirical support, references to high-risk groups permeate recent studies and reports on TASER technology.

High-risk group theory appears to derive from a compilation of findings in morbidity and mortality studies related to the use of TASER ECDs. In the earliest such study, Kornblum and Reddy (1991) examined 16 deaths proximate to the use of early generation TASER ECDs. All the deaths involved young males with a history of controlled substance abuse. Thirteen of them were under the influence of cocaine, phencyclidine (PCP), or amphetamine at the time of their death. In 11 cases, the medical examiner determined that the cause of death was an overdose of drugs. Many studies followed linking sudden deaths to the use of TASER ECDs and the use of commonly abused recreational drugs, specifically amphetamines, cocaine, lysergic acid diethylamide (LSD), marijuana, opiates, and PCP. Throughout the rest of the text, the term drug refers to one or more of these six drugs.

As the United Kingdom contemplated adopting the use of TASER ECDs, the Defence Scientific Advisory Council Sub-committee on the Medical Implications of Less-Lethal Weapons (DOMILL) (2002) issued a statement on their research. DOMILL stated that there was no experimental evidence that the use of drugs increased the susceptibility of the heart to the use of TASER ECDs. However, DOMILL also stated that there was sufficient indication from existing forensic data and known electrophysiological characteristics of the heart to opine that people intoxicated with drugs and alcohol or those with pre-existing heart disease could be more prone to adverse effects from TASER ECDs compared to unimpaired individuals.

Four years later, during evaluation of a pilot program, DOMILL (2006) issued another statement recommending that research should be undertaken to clarify potential hazards associated with the use of TASER ECDs on individuals who could be considered to have a greater risk of adverse effects. The hazards, in DOMILL's view, included the following: possible cardiac hyper susceptibility arising from drugs, acidosis, pre-existing disease, and the vulnerability of pacemakers and other implantable devices.

In 2005, the Office of the Chief Coroner for Ontario reviewed all known TASER ECD-proximate deaths in Canada to determine whether a causal relationship was present. In every case studied, coroners or medical examiners determined that the deaths were either a consequence of drug toxicity or complications of delirium rather than the result of use of TASER ECDs (Lucas and Cairns, 2006). Nonetheless, the study reinforced the correlation between the use of drugs and sudden deaths following the application of ECDs.

Ederheimer, Warner, Johnson, and Fridell (2006) conducted a study to compare characteristics of TASER ECD uses that resulted in deaths and uses that did not result in deaths. They contacted 96 agencies in 26 states and collected data on 78 deaths. They also collected data on 662 ECD non-death incidents that occurred between 2001 and 2005 in Seattle, Washington, and Madison, Wisconsin. Their analysis indicated that death incidents were more likely to involve older people, people who manifested signs of mental illness, and people under the influence of drugs.

In an examination of 37 autopsy reports of patients who had died proximate to the use of a TASER ECD, Strote and Hutson (2006) reported cardiovascular disease in 54.1 percent of the cases. They also noted the use of illegal substances in 78.4 percent of cases, and they reported a diagnosis of excited delirium in 75.7 percent of the deaths. Excited delirium is a condition manifesting as a combination of delirium, psychomotor agitation, anxiety, hallucinations, speech disturbances, disorientation, violent and bizarre behavior, insensitivity to pain, elevated body temperature, and extraordinary strength.

Vilke, Johnson, Castillo, Ederheimer, Sloan, and Chan (2006) conducted an extensive survey of police agencies that had reported a death following the application of a TASER ECD, and they collected data on 77 deaths. Autopsy reports were available for 69 individuals. Based on medical examiners' reports, alcohol and drugs were present in 29.8 percent and 76.6 percent of the subjects, respectively.

Drawing on the results of these studies, researchers began to reference attributes of narcotics use, heart disease, the presence of pacemakers and implantable defibrillating devices (ICDs), excited delirium, age, mental illness, and alcohol as indicators of vulnerable or high-risk groups. In their second report on TASER technology, Amnesty International voiced concern over what they termed the paucity of research with respect to "high risk groups such as those who have taken illicit drugs or who have underlying heart conditions (Amnesty International, 2006:28)." They also expressed concerns about ECD use on "vulnerable groups, such as children, the disabled, pregnant women and people with mental illnesses. . . (Amnesty International, 2006:28)."

In their report on mortality studies of nearly 300 TASER ECD-related deaths, the United States Department of Justice task force reported that purported safety margins of ECD deployments on healthy adults might not be applicable to "small children, those with diseased hearts, the elderly, those who are pregnant and other at-risk individuals (National Institute of Justice, 2008:4)." The task force noted that understanding of the effects of TASER ECD application in those populations was limited and that more data collection was necessary. Nonetheless, they urged that officers should avoid using ECDs against those populations. Ryan (2008) also concluded that many of the people who died in the United States had been drug-affected or were mentally ill.

The Maryland Attorney General's Task Force on Electronic Weapons recommended that law enforcement agencies should adopt use-of-force models that recognize populations at a heightened risk of

death. They listed those populations as persons with known heart conditions including pacemakers, elderly persons or young children, frail
persons or persons with very thin statures, women known to be pregnant, persons in mental/medical crisis, or persons under the influence of
drugs or intoxicated by alcohol (Higginbotham, et al., 2009).

In his report on TASER ECD use in British Columbia, Braidwood
(2009) recommended against using the ECD in medically high-risk
situations. Included in his definition of high-risk situations was deployment in any mode against an emotionally disturbed person, an elderly person, a person who the officer has reason to believe is pregnant,
or a person who the officer has reason to believe has a medical condition that may be worsened because of the deployment, such as heart
disease or an implanted pacemaker or defibrillator.

White and Ready (2009) examined media reports of TASER ECD
incidents to compare incidents in which a fatality occurred to incidents
in which a fatality did not occur. They found that suspects who were
under the influence of drugs were four times more likely to die, and
suspects who were emotionally disturbed or who were mentally ill were
nearly twice as likely to die. They found that a suspect under the influence of alcohol was less likely to die, and they reported that the age of
the suspect was not statistically significant.

The Corruption and Crime Commission (2010), the oversight body for
the Western Australia police force, released a report that criticized police
officers for using TASER ECDs against people in high-risk groups. The
Commission defined high-risk groups as individuals with a mental illness,
those who were suffering from drug and substance abuse, and those who
otherwise exhibited signs of extreme psychological distress.

The Police Executive Research Forum and the U.S. Department of
Justice (2011) jointly published guidelines for the use of TASER ECDs
noting some populations that could be at heightened risk for serious
injury or death following application of an ECD. They defined those
populations as pregnant women, elderly people, young children, visibly
frail people or people with a slight build, people with known heart conditions, people in medical or mental crisis, and people under the influence of drugs or alcohol. They recommended that police personnel
should receive training in the medical complications that might follow
the use of an ECD. They added that police officers should also be
aware that certain individuals, such as those in a state of delirium,

might be at a heightened risk for serious injury or death when subjected to ECD application or other uses of force to subdue them.

Heretofore, as the examples above illustrate, high-risk group theory has only been partially constructed. With information compiled from previous studies and reports, it is now possible to propose a more complete formulation. High-risk group theory postulates that elderly people, young children, people with pre-existing cardiovascular disease, people with pacemakers and implantable cardioverter-defibrillators (ICD), people under the influence of drugs or with a history of drug abuse, people intoxicated from alcohol or with a history of chronic alcohol abuse, people under extreme psychological distress or who exhibit signs of excited delirium, people who are mentally ill or taking psychotropic medications, people subjected to repeated or multiple applications, and pregnant women are at a heightened risk of serious injury or death following application of a TASER ECD.

Recurring references in studies and reports have led some researchers to the conclusion that high-risk group theory is well established (Ryan, 2011; Starmer and Gordon, 2007). However, oft-repeated declaration does not equate to a well-established finding regarding the higher lethality of the TASER ECD when compared to other means of subduing such high-risk individuals. What the extant literature fails to consider is that the same physiological attributes that are presumed to render members of high-risk groups more vulnerable to serious injury or death following application of a TASER ECD might render these same people more vulnerable to serious injury or death regardless of the tactics or weapons that officers use to subdue them in affecting an arrest. If that hypothesis is correct, *arguendo*, the use of TASER ECDs on people in high-risk groups is irrelevant to the rates of arrest-related sudden deaths.

DEFINING ARREST-RELATED SUDDEN DEATH

Most studies on arrest-related deaths examine police practices and policies, not the cause of death. Moreover, few studies on arrest-related deaths define exactly what arrest-related means. Unfortunately, most studies tend to include any death that happens during arrest, transport, or custody, a fact which makes it difficult to determine whether the cause of death results from factors present only during the arrest, by factors present only during the term of confinement, or by both. Consequently, police administrators have relatively little guidance on formulating use-of-force policy, in training officers to apply the appropriate quantum of force, and in instructing detectives how best to investigate arrest-related sudden deaths. The result is frequent criticism in the media, loss of trust in the community, and rising costs in defending wrongful death or excessive force lawsuits.

In a study of TASER ECD-proximate deaths, Vilke, Johnson, Castillo, Ederheimer, Sloan, and Chan (2006) include any death that occurs at a police scene or while the deceased is in police custody and an officer fires an ECD at any time during the incident. However, that definition includes the death of a prisoner who has been in confinement for months or even years following the original arrest or detention. Within that period, a number of factors post-arrest become pertinent. Detention officers might use an ECD months after commencement of detention or imprisonment, and medical conditions that did not exist at the time of the arrest could arise during the term of an individual's confinement. Vilke's definition is, therefore, overly broad for a study of arrest-related sudden deaths.

Grant, Southall, Fowler, Thomas, and Kinlock (2007), in a study of autopsy reports of 202 in-custody deaths, determined that data on the length of time an individual was in custody before death occurred were not consistently available. Therefore, they excluded any consideration of time in custody from the analysis. Ignoring such post-arrest factors as time in custody reduces the value of the study for understanding the arrest-related effects of the ECD.

Southall, Grant, Fowler, and Scott (2008) were more restrictive in their study of 45 police custody deaths. Although they did not specify a time, they included only deaths that occurred during police/citizen encounters, including field interrogations, arrest procedures, and detention. They excluded deaths resulting from suicidal hangings, police shootings and police-related motor vehicle incidents. Once more, however, the fact of including deaths in detention extends consideration of factors well after the arrest.

In 2000, Congress passed the Death in Custody Reporting Act (Public Law 106-297), a statute which required all states to submit to the Bureau of Justice Statistics (BJS) a record of any death that occurs in the process of arrest as a condition of receiving federal correctional grants. Congress left it to the BJS to define "in the process of arrest."

The BJS defines death "in the process of arrest" as all deaths of persons in the physical custody or under the physical restraint of law enforcement officers. The definition includes arrests for criminal charges and detentions for mental health issues and medical transports. The BJS includes any deaths of persons arrested or subject to arrest who dies: (1) as a result of use of force by law enforcement officers; (2) as a result of suicides, provided that law enforcement officers were in contact with the subject prior to the suicide; and (3) at medical facilities due to injuries or medical problems, including persons who die in transit from an arrest scene in a police vehicle or ambulance. The BJS excludes from the definition: (1) deaths of any other persons not subject to an attempted arrest, including bystanders and law enforcement officers killed during an attempted arrest; and (2) vehicular accident deaths that are not specifically related to arrest activities (Mumola, 2007).

Not all deaths from factors related to an arrest are immediate. Some deaths related to attributes of high-risk groups occur shortly after the arrest or detention. Therefore, it is necessary to permit consideration of deaths that occur within a reasonable time after the initial arrest. **A period of 24 hours appears consistent with other studies and medical definitions.** The World Health Organization, a specialized agency of the United Nations that acts as a coordinating authority on international public health, compiles the *International Classification of Diseases*. This document defines sudden death as cardiorespiratory collapse that occurs within 24 hours of the beginning of symptoms. In their study of TASER ECD-proximate deaths, Ederheimer, et al. (2006), include deaths that occur within 24 hours of the application of the ECD. Strote and Hutson (2009) call for a national database of deaths occurring within 24 hours of ECD use to identify cases and to better define what impact ECD use has, if any, in arrest-related deaths.

RESEARCH QUESTION

Thus far, research has not directly addressed the question of whether the use of the TASER ECD is more likely to result in death to high-risk individuals when compared to other tactics officers use to subdue or control someone who is non-compliant. It is not possible fully to answer the question of whether the use of a TASER ECD differs from other less-lethal weapons and tactics in its physiological effects on people in theoretical high-risk groups. A random clinical trial is necessary to establish causal relationships, but a clinical trial requires experimentation on the mentally ill, people intoxicated on alcohol, people intoxicated on drugs, and people with known serious cardiovascular disease. Such experimentation is ethically impermissible.

A retrospective study of all use of force incidents to compare fatal and non-fatal encounters is also unlikely. In fatal cases, autopsy reports document the physiological attributes of the deceased. Non-fatal cases, however, pose two major problems. First, in non-fatal cases current medical information is seldom available because the person did not receive injuries sufficiently serious to warrant medical treatment. Second, even when current medical records do exist, Title II of the Health Insurance Portability and Accountability Act of 1996 (Public Law 104-191) establishes policies, procedures and guidelines for maintaining the privacy and security of individually identifiable health information. Thus, those records are not available for review, except under highly limited circumstances.

It is possible, however, to compare differences in the physiological attributes and mental health histories of arrest-related sudden deaths by examining autopsy reports of the deceased. One can then estimate whether a significant difference exists in high-risk group attributes between deaths proximate to the use of a TASER ECD and deaths proximate to the use of other less-lethal weapons and tactics.

A retrospective case study approach limits the questions the research can answer. *This study seeks to determine whether attributes of high-risk group theory appear more often in TASER ECD-proximate deaths than in other arrest-related sudden deaths not involving an ECD.* If, as high-risk group theory predicts, people with nominal high-risk group attributes are more susceptible to sudden death following application of a TASER ECD, then one should expect to find those attributes more often in ECD-proximate deaths than in non-ECD arrest-related deaths.

To answer the research question, one must identify and define differences between TASER ECD-proximate deaths and non-ECD deaths related to the following attributes: *age, cardiovascular disease,* the presence of a *pacemaker or ICD,* the presence of *drugs* in the body of the deceased or a *history of drug abuse*, the presence of *alcohol* in the body of the deceased or a *history of chronic alcohol abuse*, evidence of *excited delirium, mental illness*, and the presence of *psychotropic medications* in the body of the deceased. The last two attributes of high-risk group theory, multiple applications of the TASER ECD and pregnancy will not be tested in this study. Because the multiple application attribute does not apply to non-ECD arrest-related sudden deaths, there is no group against which to compare, and, as will be discussed in the literature review, there is no known case of a pregnant woman dying following application of a TASER ECD.

CHAPTER 2

What We Know About Arrest-Related Sudden Death

Limits on available data inhibit researchers from determining the physiological impacts of TASER ECDs on arrest-related sudden deaths at the incident level. Optimally, researchers could draw on a reliable, systematic national database of incident-level data on all uses of force and their associated outcomes. However, no such database exists (Ho, 2009; White and Ready, 2010). Additionally, there is no nationwide data collection system to collect reliable and systematic incident-level data on arrest-related deaths. All five major data sources for examining in-custody deaths have substantial limitations (Borrego, 2011; White, et al., 2013). These sources include the FBI's Supplemental Homicide Report, the Bureau of Justice Statistics Deaths in Custody Reporting Program (DCRP), and the Center for Disease Control's National Violent Death Reporting System (NVDRS), Web-Based Injury Statistics Query and Reporting System (WISQRS) and Wide-Ranging Online Data for Epidemiologic Research (WODER).

Therefore, it is necessary to examine a range of literature and data to investigate whether elderly people, young children, people with pre-existing cardiovascular disease, people with pacemakers and ICDs, people under the influence of drugs or with a history of drug abuse, people intoxicated from alcohol or with a history of chronic alcohol abuse, people under extreme psychological distress or who exhibit signs of excited delirium, or people who are mentally ill or taking psychotropic medications, are at a heightened risk of death following application of a TASER ECD.

SUDDEN IN-CUSTODY DEATH SYNDROME

Since the 1990s, medical and criminal justice research has identified a relatively consistent constellation of factors that appear to increase the likelihood of arrest-related sudden death: physical struggle, the use of drugs, restraint aids, and natural disease (Grant, et al., 2007). In some instances, however, post-mortem and toxicological examinations fail to produce a definitive diagnosis. The lack of an identifiable anatomical cause occasionally leads pathologists, medical examiners, and coroners to attribute death in such cases to sudden in-custody death syndrome (Robison and Hunt, 2005).

Much of the discussion and debate regarding in-custody deaths seek to assign a single cause rather than to consider clusters of symptoms and behaviors (Ho, 2005). Legal reasoning favors single proximate causes rather than complex medical conditions, and popular media favor controversy and blame rather than balance and explanation (Farnham and Kennedy, 1997). In many sudden in-custody deaths, the deceased has no history of prior illnesses or significant underlying medical conditions. Such sudden and unexpected custody deaths often occur during the process of arrest, or very soon after confrontation with law enforcement officers, and that propinquity leads to assumptions that police tactics and/or weapons are somehow to blame.

Sudden in-custody death cases share many similarities and patterns. First, an individual often presents in a state of agitation or delirium resulting from mental illness or from the use of stimulants or other drugs. Second, the individual exhibits aggressive or violent tendencies that require officers to employ various force options to subdue him or her. Third, the individual suddenly becomes quiet, calm, and unresponsive. Shortly thereafter, officers note that the individual is not breathing and is in cardiopulmonary arrest for which resuscitation efforts are futile. Fourth, on autopsy, there is often no clear anatomical or toxicological explanation for the death (Chan, 2006). Medical literature on sudden in-custody death syndrome recalls that such cases closely mimic deaths of institutionalized mental health patients dating back to the mid-1800s (Ho, 2005).

It is important to note that the constellation of factors related to sudden in-custody death syndrome can affect an individual before, during, and after police intervention. The complex chain of events leading to death often begins long before law enforcement involvement. The most recent event in that chain or some highly notable event in that chain, such as police intervention and the use of force, is not necessarily the cause of or a significant contributing factor to the death (Ho, 2005). A grand jury in Miami-Dade, Florida, after investigating a series of arrest-related deaths, reported that the causes of death listed in autopsy reports for people who died after being shocked with a TASER ECD were similar to one another. Additionally, the causes of death listed for people who died after being shocked with a TASER ECD were similar to the causes of death listed on the autopsy reports of non-ECD arrest-related deaths (Recinos, Miller, Hutchinson, Llanes, Acosta, Alayon, Armesto, Campbell-Dumeus, Diblin, Edgington, Fajardo, Geroges, Laurenceau, Llama, Lopez, Pruss, Ramos, Robinette, Santos, and Thomas, 2005).

SUDDEN CARDIAC DEATH

Sudden cardiac death is a major topic for research and debate regarding the use of TASER ECDs. Many arrest-related sudden deaths occur in individuals with no history of heart disease. Yet, pathologists often diagnose the cause of death as having cardiac etiology, which leads some to argue that the electrical current of the ECD must have had some adverse effect on the cardiac muscle. However, sudden cardiac death long predates the use of ECDs, and it is a common phenomenon. Sudden cardiac death, commonly known as cardiac arrest, is the unexpected and abrupt loss of heart function in a person who may or who may not have previously diagnosed heart disease. The time and mode of death are unexpected, but death can occur instantly or very shortly after the first symptoms appear.

When the definition of sudden death is restricted to deaths occurring less than two hours from the onset of symptoms, 12 percent of all natural deaths are sudden, and 88 percent of those sudden deaths are due to cardiac disease. In autopsy-based studies, pathologists report cardiac etiology in 60 to 70 percent of sudden death victims (Pinto and Josephson, 2004). The annual incidence of sudden cardiac death in the United States alone is approximately 460,000 cases and, although the absolute risk is greater in cardiac high-risk populations, many sudden cardiac deaths occur in patients who were not previously identified as being at risk. Sudden cardiac death is the first symptom of cardiovascular disease in approximately 25 percent of patients (Cronin, 2012), and in about 50 percent of sudden cardiac deaths with structurally normal hearts sudden death is the very first manifestation of heart disease (Chugh, Kelly, and Titus, 2000).

Several clinical and autopsy-based studies report the triggering of sudden cardiac death with exercise. Data supporting the theory that vigorous physical activity can trigger VF come from emergency medical records. In one review carried out in Seattle, 11 percent of 316 consecutive victims died during or immediately after vigorous physical exercise. Researchers estimated the incidence of exercise-related sudden death at 5.4 deaths per 100,000 people. In Miami, 17 percent of 150 consecutive patients who died in the emergency department of a local hospital suffered exertion-related sudden death (Pinto and Josephson, 2004). The incidence of sudden cardiac death during vigorous activity versus the incidence of sudden cardiac death during sedentary activity is five times higher for men who exercise frequently, and 56 times higher for men who exercise infrequently (Fletcher, Flipse, and Oken, 2004). Clearly, the risk of sudden cardiac death following violent exertion, such as a struggle with police or straining against restraints, increases many times for people with or without preexisting cardiovascular disease, regardless of the tactic or weapon an officer used.

Not all sudden cardiac deaths have a cause that can be determined at autopsy. As many as 30 percent of sudden cardiac deaths involve previously healthy children, adolescents, and young adults with no identifiable abnormalities found at autopsy (Carturan, Tester, Brost, Basso, Thiene, and Ackerman, 2008). In a study of approximately 852,300 women who entered basic military training over the period 1977 to 2001, Eckart, Scoville, Shry, Potter, and Tedrow (2006) found that sudden death with a structurally normal heart was the leading cause of death in female recruits. In a review of clinical and autopsy records of 19 sudden cardiac deaths that occurred among more than 1.6 million Air Force recruits during basic training between 1965 and 1985, pathologists identified no anatomic cause of death in three of the cases (Phillips, Robinowitz, Higgins, Boran, Reed, and Virmani, 1986). Inherited electrophysiological abnormalities, known as primary electrical diseases, are often the common underlying cause of many sudden unexplained cardiac deaths (Estes, 2005). These abnormalities are often undiagnosed before death, and are not apparent at autopsy.

DEMOGRAPHIC FACTORS

Research on the correlation of demographic factors, such as age, sex, and ethnicity, to arrest-related deaths are rare. However, many studies investigating other correlations report findings on demographic factors. Because the results are reported so differently across studies, particularly as they relate to age and race, it is difficult to interpret them consistently.

Age

In studies on arrest-related deaths, ages of the deceased range from 15 to 75 years (Ho, 2009). The mean age is 35.7 years (Ho, Heegaard, Dawes, Matarajan, Reardon, and Miner, 2009; Southall, et al., 2008), and 54.6 percent of the deceased are between 25 and 44 years (Burch, 2011). Reports regarding age in studies related to deaths proximate to the use of a TASER ECD differ little from reports of age in studies of all arrest-related deaths. Researchers report ages of the deceased range from 17 to 65 years (Williams, 2008). Mean ages range from 34.8 years (Strote, Campbell, Pease, Hamman, and Hutson, 2005) to 35.9 years (White, et al., 2013). Approximately 65.9 percent of deaths proximate to the use of a TASER ECD are between 21 and 40 years of age (White, et al., 2013).

Reports on the use of TASER ECDs, regardless of whether a death occurred, list a range from 9 years of age (Angelidis, Basta, Walsh, Hutson, and Strote, 2009) to 80 years of age (Bozeman, et al., 2009). The mean ages in those reports range from 30 years (Eastman, Metzger, Pepe, Benitez, Decker, Rinnert, Field, and Friese, 2008) to 32 years (Bozeman, et al., 2009). In a study of consecutive uses of TASER ECDs that included 100 cases of people 17 years of age or younger, the range was 13 years to 17 years, and the mean age was 16.1 years (Gardner, Hauda, and Bozeman, 2012).

Sex

Arrest data from the FBI's UCR from 2003 through 2009 indicate that 75.9 percent of all arrests were male, and 24.1 percent of all arrests were female (Burch, 2011). Statistics on arrest-related deaths yield vastly different ratios. According to the DCRP, from 2003 through 2009 95.4 percent of arrest-related deaths were men, and 4.5 percent were women. The sex in 0.1 percent of those deaths was unknown or was not reported (Burch, 2011). Studies related to arrest-related deaths report that the percentages of deaths of men range from 93.3 percent (Southall, et al., 2008) to 96.3 percent (Ho, Heegaard, et al., 2009).

The range is much wider for reports on uses of TASER ECDs regardless of whether a death occurs. Males comprise from 85.1 percent (Gau, Mosher, and Pratt, 2010) to 93.7 percent (Bozeman, Barnes, Winslow, Johnson, Phillips, and Alson, 2009) of subjects on whom officers apply an ECD. However, in studies of TASER ECD-proximate deaths, the percentages of deaths of males is much higher and more closely aligned with data on all arrest-related deaths, ranging from 95.8 percent (Williams, 2008) to 97.4 percent (White, et al., 2013). None of the studies purports to explain the disparity in the rates of female arrestees compared to arrest-related deaths of females.

Race/Ethnicity

Studies on arrest-related deaths or on the use of TASER ECDs seldom report race and ethnicity data, but a few studies give some indication of the racial and ethnic composition of cases studied. In a study of 45 arrest-related deaths in Maryland, Southall, et al. (2008) report that 80 percent of the deaths involved Blacks. The rest they described as mostly White, but there was no further breakdown of the data. The BJS reported that Whites constituted 42.1 percent of arrest-related deaths reported to the DCRP over the period 2003 to 2009, 31.8 percent were Black, 19.7 percent were Hispanic, and the remaining 6.4 percent were classified as other (Burch, 2011).

In a study involving one state patrol agency in one unidentified state, Gau, et al. (2010) reported that 72.3 percent of those who received a TASER ECD application were White, 8.9 percent were Black, 11.7 percent were Hispanic, and 7.1 percent were other races. Williams (2008), in a study of 213 TASER ECD-proximate deaths nationwide from 1983 through 2005, reported that the race and ethnicity of those who died closely resembled the race and ethnicity of the arrest-related deaths reported in the DCRP. Whites comprised 40.4 percent of the deaths, Blacks were 37.1 percent, Hispanics were 17.8 percent, and the rest, categorized as other, comprised the remaining 4.7 percent.

ALCOHOL AND DRUGS

A principal premise of high-risk group theory is that people who are intoxicated from alcohol or drugs are more susceptible to adverse effects following the use of a TASER ECD. It is well documented in medical literature that deaths from misuse and abuse of alcohol and drugs are common. Alcohol is the most commonly abused drug in the United States, and drugs most commonly used for recreational purposes include cocaine, methamphetamine and amphetamine derivatives, and cannabis (Milroy and Parai, 2011).

In a study of 213 TASER ECD-proximate deaths, Williams (2008) found that, in 125 deaths that occurred nationwide between 2001 and 2005 for which autopsy and toxicology reports were available, 98 (78.4 percent) had positive results for alcohol, drugs, or both in their systems at the time of their deaths. Fox and Payne-James (2012) studied 175 deaths proximate to the application of a TASER ECD. Of those cases, 108 (61.7 percent) involved intoxication from alcohol or drugs. In a study of 392 arrest-related deaths following the application of a TASER ECD, White, et al. (2013) found that in 53.5 percent of the cases the deceased were intoxicated from alcohol and/or drugs during their encounter with the police. Medical literature makes clear, however, that people who are intoxicated from alcohol or drugs are at greater risk of sudden death even absent police intervention.

Alcohol

Years of research clearly demonstrate the deleterious effects of heavy alcohol consumption. Several case history studies suggest that chronic alcoholics can suffer from atrial fibrillation, an irregularity in heartbeat caused by involuntary contractions of small areas of heart-wall muscle, and VT even in the absence of clinical heart disease (Kupari and Koskinin, 1998). The literature also demonstrates a statistically significant correlation between consumption of more than five drinks per day with an increased risk of sudden cardiac death (Dyer, Stamler, Paul, Berkson, Lepper, McKean, Shekelle, Lindberg, and Garside, 1977; Wannamethee and Shaper, 1992).

The effects of acute alcohol intoxication are no less grave. Complications of acute intoxication include cardiomyopathy (a disease of the heart muscle), arrhythmias, ketoacidosis (a metabolic state associated with high concentrations of ketone bodies), and acute respiratory distress, all of which can lead to sudden cardiac death (Al-Sanouri, Dikin, and Soubani, 2005).

Studies regarding moderate consumption of alcohol produce decidedly different findings. People who consume two to four drinks per week have a 60 percent reduced risk of sudden cardiac death, and those who consume five to six drinks per week have a 79 percent reduced risk of sudden cardiac death compared with people who rarely or never consume alcohol (Albert, Manson, Cook, Ajani, Gaziano, and Hennekens, 1999).

In a study of 213 TASER ECD-proximate deaths, Williams (2008) found that, in 125 deaths that occurred between 2001 and 2005 for which autopsy and toxicology reports were available, 20 (16.0 percent) had positive results for alcohol. In their study of 175 deaths proximate to the application of a TASER ECD, Fox and Payne-James (2012) found that nine (5.1 percent) were intoxicated from alcohol at the time of their deaths.

In the only human model experiment testing the effects of TASER technology on intoxicated subjects, no clinically significant effects on markers of acidosis or cardiac injury were detected in 22 people who had a minimum blood alcohol concentration of 0.08 milligrams per deciliter (mg/dL), and who then experienced a 15-second discharge from an X26 (Moscati, Ho, Dawes, and Miner 2010). The literature lacks any alcohol-specific experiments on ECD application in acutely intoxicated animal models (Moscati and Ho, 2009).

Cocaine
Cocaine is second only to cannabis as the most widely trafficked illicit drug in the world (Milroy and Parai, 2011). As the use of cocaine increases in the United States, the number of cocaine-related cardiovascular events, including sudden death, increases commensurately (Lange and Hillis, 2010). Cocaine is a sympathomimetic agent that activates centrally and peripherally the sympathetic nervous system, that part of the autonomic nervous system that is active during stress or danger and is involved in regulating pulse and blood pressure, dilating pupils, and changing muscle tone (Gunn, Evans, and Kriger, 2009). People with high blood concentrations of cocaine exhibit a typical pattern of symptoms with agitation, followed by confusion, seizures, and a rise in core body temperature (Karch and Stephens, 1999). The presence of hyperthermia, a core body temperature higher than 103°F, is strongly indicative of a cocaine-induced event (Stephens, Jentzen, Karch, Wetli, and Mash, 2004).

The use of cocaine, chronic and acute, has profound effects on the cardiovascular system, and it is a common cause of sudden death (Milroy and Parai, 2011). Cocaine acts as a vasoconstrictor that elevates blood pressure, constricts coronary arteries, and reduces blood supply to the heart. High doses of cocaine can produce cardiac arrhythmias and sudden death by slowing nerve impulse conduction by blocking the movement of sodium ions in cardiac channels (Crumb and Clarkson, 1990).

Post-mortem estimation of the time and quantity of cocaine ingested does not reliably predict toxicity or lethality because post-mortem cocaine levels do not necessarily correlate to drug toxicity or poisoning, and lethal levels of cocaine are not necessary to trigger cardiovascular events (Stephens, et al., 2004). The concurrent use of alcohol and cocaine produces a new compound, cocaethylene, which lasts longer in the body and has even more potent toxic effects than either cocaine or alcohol alone (Sztajnkrycer and Baez, 2005).

Of the 175 TASER ECD-proximate deaths in the study by Fox and Payne-James (2012), 37.7 percent had toxicology results positive for the presence of cocaine. Of the 125 deaths for which autopsy and toxicology reports were available in the Williams study, 47.2 percent had positive results for cocaine, its metabolite, benzoylecgonine, or its ethyl ester, ethylbenzoylecgonine (Williams, 2008).

In the only animal model experiment of the effects of cocaine on TASER technology, Lakkireddy, Wallick, Ryschon, Chung, Butany, Martin, Saliba, Kowalewski, Natale, and Tchou (2006) found that infusion of cocaine into five pigs increased ECD cardiac safety margins by 50 to 100 percent above baseline safety margins, thereby decreasing the risk of an adverse cardiac effect. Applying sufficient voltage to a heart cell opens its sodium-ion channels and starts contractions. Counter intuitively, cocaine blocks the voltage-activated sodium channels, making it more difficult for electricity to trigger a muscle contraction (Tchou, 2007). There are no human model experiments on the effects of cocaine on TASER technology.

Methamphetamine and Amphetamine Derivatives
Amphetamines have a long history of abuse and are clearly associated with increased risks of cardiovascular complications such as stroke and myocardial infarction (MI), the death of a segment of heart muscle (Dawson and Moffat, 2012). Methamphetamine has effects similar to cocaine on the cardiovascular system, with the hearts of chronic users showing hypertrophy, growth in size of the heart through an increase in the size of its cells, and microvascular disease, which are diseases in

the finer blood vessels, including capillaries. Use of 3,4-methylene-dioxy-N-methamphetamine (MDMA), an amphetamine derivative better known as ecstasy, results in similar cardiovascular changes (Milroy and Parai, 2011).

Methamphetamine is an indirect sympathomimetic agent distinguished from amphetamine by a more rapid distribution into the central nervous system. It is associated with adverse effects to every organ system, although the most significant morbidity and mortality occur because of cardiovascular effects (Vearrier, Greenberg, Miller, Okaneku, and Haggerty, 2012). Users have significantly higher rates of coronary artery disease than the public. Even patients with normal coronary arteries are at risk for methamphetamine-induced MI, which can result in cardiogenic shock (an inadequate circulation of blood due to primary failure of the ventricles of the heart to function effectively) leading to death (Vearrier, et al., 2012).

Experimental evidence suggests that MDMA has cardiotoxic properties similar to cocaine and methamphetamine. Users of MDMA appear to be at risk similar to users of other stimulants for myocardial hypertrophy and cardiotoxicity, a drug-induced suppression of heart muscle or its conduction system (Patel, Belson, Wright, Lub, Heningere, and Miller, 2005).

Fox and Payne-James (2012) studied 175 deaths proximate to the application of a TASER ECD and found that 25 of those cases involved methamphetamine and two involved MDMA, a total of 15.4 percent. In a study of 213 TASER ECD-proximate deaths, Williams (2008) found that, in 125 deaths that occurred between 2001 and 2005 for which autopsy and toxicology reports were available, 32 cases, or 25.6 percent, had positive results for amphetamine, methamphetamine, or MDMA.

Dawes, Ho, Cole, Reardon, Lundin, Terwey, Falvey, and Miner (2010) infused four sheep with 0.5 mg of methamphetamine per kg of body weight, four received 1.0 mg/kg, four received 1.5 mg/kg, and four control group animals received no methamphetamine. They found that in eight animals weighing less than 32 kg, application of a TASER ECD triggered cardiac capture, a beating of the heart in response to an external electrical stimulus. In eight animals weighing more than 32 kg, however, there was no such effect. In no case did the application of a TASER ECD produce VF. There are no human model experiments on the effects of methamphetamine on TASER technology.

Cannabis

Reports linking cannabis use to MI and sudden cardiac death first appeared in the late 1970s (Karch, 2006). Medical literature has reported cases of acute coronary ischemia, an inadequate supply of blood and oxygen to meet the metabolic demands of the heart muscle, even with normal coronary arteries. The literature is undecided on whether cannabis use causes coronary artery disease (Lindsay, Foale, Warren, and Henry, 2005). There have also been several case reports suggesting that marijuana can trigger MI and arrhythmias (Karch, 2006). Although rare, sudden death has been reported in cannabis users with and without evidence of coronary heart disease, and the risk of MI within an hour following cannabis use is 4.8 times higher than the risks for non-users (Lindsay, et al, 2005).

In a study of 213 TASER ECD-proximate deaths, Williams (2008) found that, in 125 deaths that occurred between 2001 and 2005 for which autopsy and toxicology reports were available, 16 (12.8 percent) were positive for marijuana. There are no experiments on the interrelationship of TASER technology and cannabis use in either animal or human models.

PCP

PCP and its derivative, ketamine, induce alterations in behavior that resemble schizophrenia, and acute ingestion of PCP can induce a schizophrenia-like state in otherwise healthy humans (Kargieman, Riga, Artigas, and Celada, 2012). These behavioral changes were first observed in the late 1950s when PCP, administered to healthy volunteers, generated a form of psychosis. When the drug was administered to schizophrenic patients it intensified their symptoms of profound disorganization. Some of these symptoms lasted for weeks. PCP psychosis was so similar to schizophrenia that many psychiatrists could not distinguish them without an indication of prior drug abuse (Olmedo, 2006). PCP was first used as an intravenous anesthetic because it did not significantly depress respiratory or cardiovascular function. However, patients developed post-anesthetic delirium and hallucinations. Violent behavior has often been attributed to the use of PCP, but the correlation between PCP and violent psychotic behavior is unclear (Pestaner and Southall, 2003).

In a study of deaths following the application of early generation TASER ECDs, Kornblum and Reddy (1991) found that 8 of 16 deaths

(50 percent) involved the use of PCP. Fox and Payne-James (2012) studied 175 deaths proximate to the application of a TASER ECD and found that 2 (1.1 percent) of those cases involved PCP. In a study of 213 TASER ECD-proximate deaths, Williams (2008) found that, in 125 deaths that occurred between 2001 and 2005 for which autopsy and toxicology reports were available, 2 cases, or 1.6 percent, had positive results for PCP. There are no experiments on the interrelationship of TASER technology and PCP use in either animal or human models.

Opiates
Opiates are a class of drugs that include opium or opium derivatives, either natural or synthetic, and have a sedative effect. Opiates include buprenorphine, codeine, diphenoxylate, fentanyl, heroin, hydrocodone, hydromorphone, levacetylmethadol, levorphanol, meperidine, methadone, morphine, morphine diacetate, opium, oxycodone, oxymorphone, propoxyphene, and tramadol. Opium, a product of the poppy plant, was cultivated as long ago as 3400 B.C. In 1806, Frederich Sertürner isolated the primary active ingredient in opium, which he named morphium. Morphium, now known as morphine, is 10 times more potent than opium itself. In 1874, chemists devised a chemical bonding process for morphine that produced heroin—a substance about three times as potent as morphine. Bayer Laboratories of Germany initially marketed heroin in 1898 as a non-addictive substitute for codeine, which is also derived from opium. It took nearly a decade to realize that heroin was the most addictive of the opiates, able to affect brain functioning faster than anything then known (Isralowitz and Myers, 2011). Recently, increased use of opiates to manage chronic pain has led to new and growing problems with addiction and misuse (Okie, 2010).

In a study of 213 TASER ECD-proximate deaths, Williams (2008) found that, in 125 deaths that occurred between 2001 and 2005 for which autopsy and toxicology reports were available, 3 cases, or 2.4 percent, had positive results for opiates. There are no experiments on the interrelationship of TASER technology and opiate use in either animal or human models.

LSD
Albert Hofmann first synthesized LSD, a semi-synthetic product of lysergic acid, in 1938. He accidentally discovered its psychological

effects in 1943. LSD was produced commercially in the 1950s as an experimental tool to enhance the effects of psychotherapeutic treatments. By the late 1960s, people began using LSD recreationally, leading to the psychedelic movement during the student protests of the era. Although the protest movement has declined, LSD has appeared as a major drug of abuse in every *National Survey on Drug Use and Health* since the 1970s (Passiel, Halpern, Stichtenoth, Enrich, and Hintzen, 2008).

Moderate doses of LSD can alter the state of consciousness characterized by euphoria and altered psychological functioning. Traumatic experiences include mood swings and rare flashback phenomena. Psychomotor functions, such as coordination and reaction time are frequently impaired after using LSD. Researchers have also noted decreases in performance on tests of attention and concentration. However, despite some cases of exceedingly high LSD concentrations, there have been no documented human deaths from an overdose (Passiel, et al., 2008). None of the studies on arrest-related deaths or TASER ECD-proximate deaths comment on any case related to the use of LSD, and there are no experiments on the interrelationship of TASER technology and LSD use in either animal or human models.

MENTAL ILLNESS

A principal tenet of high-risk group theory is that people with mental illness are especially susceptible to sudden arrest-related death following application of a TASER ECD. However, no one has ever described a mechanism to explain how or why. There is evidence in medical literature to demonstrate that populations with mental illnesses, particularly schizophrenia, are at higher risk for sudden death (Glassman and Bigger, 2001). The death rate for the mentally ill is nearly three times higher than the death rate for the general population due to an increased suicide rate and increased mortality due to natural causes, including cardiovascular disease (Haddad and Anderson, 2002).

Additionally, medical literature indicates that the taking of antipsychotic drugs to treat mental illness increases the rate of sudden death. Although it is difficult to be sure that a specific drug is at fault in a patient population that is already more likely to experience sudden death, the first report of sudden arrhythmic death related to the use of an antipsychotic drug appeared in 1963 (Glassman and Bigger, 2001). Recent studies indicate that current use of antipsychotic drugs is associated with a higher risk of sudden cardiac death, but the risks are also elevated with long-term use (Sabine, Straus, Bleumink, Dieleman, van der Lei, Jong, Kingma, Sturkenboom, and Stricker, 2004). Patients using antipsychotics have 1.7 to 5.3 times higher rates of cardiac arrest or ventricular arrhythmias than controls (Koponen, Alaräisänen, Saari, Pelkonen, Huikuri, Raatikainen, Savolainen, and Isohanni, 2008). Ray, Chung, Murray, Hall, and Stein (2009), in a long-term observational study of Medicaid enrollees in Tennessee, found that the risk of sudden death for individuals receiving antipsychotic drugs was almost 2.4 times greater than for nonusers.

Research reveals that the use of antipsychotics can cause sudden death through several mechanisms, but particular interest centers on torsade de pointes (TdP), a polymorphic ventricular arrhythmia that can progress from QT prolongation (delayed repolarization of the heart following a heartbeat) to VF and sudden cardiac death (Haddad and Anderson, 2002). The QT interval runs from the beginning of the QRS complex to the end of the T-wave, and it represents the time between the onset of electrical depolarization of the ventricles and the end of depolarization. QT prolongation is a marker for the development of TdP, and prolongation longer than 100 milliseconds (ms) might be a risk factor for life-threatening ventricular arrhythmias (Haddad and Anderson, 2002).

Little literature exists regarding the implications of TASER ECD use on individuals with mental illness (O'Brien, McKenna, and Simpson, 2007). In a study on the use of ECDs in New Zealand, O'Brien, McKenna, Thom, Diesfeld, and Simpson (2011) discovered that officers were more than twice as likely to discharge TASER ECDs in mental health emergencies as in criminal arrests, but they found no deaths or long-term health implications in the mentally ill population. In a study of the Critical Incident Team of the Akron (Ohio) Police Department, researchers examined the use of a TASER ECD on 27 individuals with a mental illness and reported no incident resulting in death or serious harm to the individuals in crisis (Munetz, Fitzgerald, and Woody, 2006).

White and Ready (2009) studied news media reports of TASER ECD incidents over the period 2002 to 2006, comparing incidents in which a fatality occurred to incidents in which a fatality did not occur. They found that a suspect was twice as likely to die following TASER ECD deployment if the suspect was emotionally disturbed or mentally ill. In a study of TASER ECD-proximate deaths, Williams (2008) found that in 125 deaths that occurred between 2001 and 2005 for which autopsy and toxicology reports were available a total of 25 (20.0 percent) had a history of mental illness.

Ho, Dawes, Johnson, Lundin, and Miner (2007) studied a database of more than 10,000 TASER ECD applications and found 2452 reports of use on mentally ill persons. The researchers discovered that in 36 of those cases the subject died within 72 hours after exposure. The researchers noted that in 32 of the 36 deaths officers reported the ECD had no effect on the subject. In 33 of the 36 cases, coroners or medical examiners concluded that the ECD was not the primary cause of death. Commonly listed causes of death included illicit drug intoxication, excited delirium, and cardiac disease. In the remaining three cases, no cause of death was available.

EXCITED DELIRIUM SYNDROME

Perhaps the most contentious and misunderstood proposition of high-risk group theory is excited delirium syndrome (ExDS). Critics of TASER technology claim that findings of ExDS as a cause of death merely excuse inappropriate or excessive use of ECDs (Amnesty International, 2008a; Braidwood, 2009; Schlosberg, 2005; Stoughton, Pendergrass, Zelon, and Al-Khatib, 2011; Whitfield and Lai, 2011). They note that the American Medical Association does not recognize ExDS, and the term does not appear in the *International Statistical Classification of Diseases and Related Health Issues, 10th Revision*, or the *Diagnostic and Statistical Manual of Mental Disorders, 4th Edition* (Ranson, 2012).

In France in 1832, L. F. Calmeil first described an uncommon but life-threatening psychosis with extreme hyperactivity and mounting fear fading to stuporous exhaustion, a complex of symptoms similar to ExDS (Morrison and Sadler, 2001). Many medical experts argue that Luther Bell, an American physician and experienced mental hospital superintendent, first diagnosed the syndrome in 1849 when he described Bell's mania, a condition in which mentally ill patients died unexpectedly following onset of specific symptoms (Bell, 1849). Emil Kraeplin, a German psychiatrist, described in 1896 a very similar set of symptoms that he called *dementia praecox* (Di Maio and Di Maio, 2006). Research in the 1930s produced several publications that described similar syndromes leading to an unexpected death. Irving Derby described the condition as manic-depressive exhaustion, G. M. Davidson labeled it acute lethal excitement, and N. R. Shulak detailed cases he referred to as excited psychotic furors (Di Maio and Di Maio, 2006).

In a review of literature on the syndrome, Kraines (1934) noted that standardized nomenclature did not yet exist. Consequently, the literature has referred to ExDS by many names over the course of 150 years: acute delirious mania, acute delirium, acute exhaustive mania, acute exhaustive psychosis, acute lethal excitement, acute psychotic furors, Bell's mania, collapse delirium, deadly catatonia, delirious mania, delirium grave, excited psychotic furors, exhaustion death, exhaustion psychosis, exhaustive syndrome, fatal catatonia, fulminating psychosis, hypertoxic schizophrenia, lethal catatonia, life-threatening psychosis, malignant catatonia, manic delirium, psychotic exhaustion, specific febrile delirium, and typhomania. ExDS is currently the commonly accepted term to describe the stereotypical constellation of psychomotor symptoms (Woodford, 2006).

Originally, ExDS referred only to cases that resulted in death, and it was closely associated with sudden in-custody death syndrome. Over time, however, the term found its way into emergency medical, psychiatric, law enforcement, prehospital, and medicolegal literature referring to cases that did not necessarily result in death (Vilke, DeBard, Chan, Ho, Dawes, Hall, Curtis, Costello, Mash, Coffman, McMullen, Metzger, Roberts, Sztajnkrycer, Henderson, Adler, Czarnecki, Heck, and Bozeman, 2011). Although research waned following the 1930s, resurgence in the 1980s marked a significant change in our collective understanding of ExDS. Wetli and Fishbain (1985) reintroduced ExDS, relating it to use of cocaine, and spurring increased research and published literature. Medical science no longer recognized ExDS only as a condition of mental illness. It had developed symptoms attributable to the use of illegal stimulant drugs, such as cocaine and methamphetamine, and to medications used to treat chronic mental illnesses (Di Maio and Di Miao, 2006).

The National Association of Medical Examiners has recognized ExDS since the 1990s (Vilke, et al., 2011), and the American College of Emergency Physicians recognized ExDS as a unique syndrome in 2009 (Hoffman, 2009). In 2008, the Minister of Justice and the Minister of Health for Nova Scotia, Canada, convened an advisory panel to review the phenomenon and its role in custody deaths. The panel concluded that there is general agreement in the scientific literature that mortality rates increase in the presence of the signs and symptoms of ExDS, even with medical intervention or in the absence of restraint by law enforcement. However, the panel preferred the term autonomic hyperarousal state to describe the cluster of symptoms (Kutcher, Ayer, Bowes, Ross, Sanford, Smith, Techan, and Theriault, 2009).

ExDS is comprised of four components, which appear in sequence: hyperthermia, delirium with agitation, respiratory arrest, and death (Wetli, Mash, and Karch, 1996). Patients exhibit bizarre and violent behavior characterized by aggression, combativeness, hyperactivity, paranoia, incoherent and undirected mental and physical aggression, and hyperthermia that often precedes fatal cardiopulmonary arrest (Roberts, 2007). Observers often describe extreme sweating, bizarre speech and behavior, extraordinary strength and seemingly limitless endurance (Farnham and Kennedy, 1997). Underlying causes of ExDS include manic-depressive psychosis, chronic schizophrenia, intoxication with sympathomimetic or anticholinergic drugs, alcohol withdrawal, and head trauma (Park, Korn, and Henderson, 2001).

Although there is no known anatomic cause of death in ExDS cases, coroners or medical examiners often cite catecholamine-induced cardiac arrhythmias (irregular cardiac rhythms caused by naturally occurring compounds in the body such as epinephrine, norepinephrine or dopamine), restraint or positional asphyxia, or adverse cardiorespiratory effects of ECDs. However, case reviews demonstrate that the individuals generally are medically unstable and in a rapidly declining state that has a high risk of mortality even with medical intervention and in the absence of restraint stress or ECD deployment (Mash, Duque, Pablo, Quin, Adi, Hearn, Hyma, Karch, Druid, and Wetli, 2009). Medical literature supports that mental stress, with or without physical exertion or underlying pathologic conditions, can cause sudden cardiac death. The forensic literature also documents sudden death during emotional experiences. Thus, it is apparent that physiologic responses to stressful psychological factors might alone provoke sudden death (Mirchandani, Rorke, Sekula-Perlman, and Hood, 1994).

In a study of 90 ExDS patients, Mash, et al. (2009) found that psychostimulants, agents that temporarily arouse or accelerate physiological or organic activity such as methamphetamine and cocaine, were present in 94 percent of the cases. The Ontario (Canada) Coroner's Office published a study of 21 cases of ExDS deaths that occurred between 1988 and 1995 within the province of Ontario (Pollanen, Chiasson, Cairns, and Young, 1998). Twelve subjects experienced ExDS caused by a psychiatric disorder, and eight subjects experienced cocaine induced psychosis. Eighteen of the deaths occurred when the victims were in police custody and could not be resuscitated. Of the 21 deaths, none followed the use of a TASER ECD. Stratton, Rogers, Brickett, and Gruzinski (2001) examined 216 arrests and detentions of subjects requiring restraint for ExDS in Los Angeles from 1992 through 1998. They found that 18 people died following restraint, but 198 subjects survived. Of the 18 deaths, 14 had stimulant drugs in their bodies. In five of the deaths, officers used a TASER ECD. In the remaining 13 deaths, officers used other force options. In each case, death was preceded by a short period during which the victim ceased struggling against restraints and developed labored or shallow breathing. In a study of 213 TASER ECD-proximate deaths, Williams (2008) found that, in 125 deaths wherein autopsy reports were available, coroners or medical examiners listed ExDS as the cause of death or as a contributing factor to the death in 44 cases.

PREGNANCY

Little is known about the effects of electrical exposure on a pregnant woman or on a fetus. Most of the literature is a collection of case series reports, and there is only one report in the medical literature directly addressing application of a first generation TASER ECD (Mehl, 1992). Neither news media nor other sources have reported a TASER ECD-proximate death of a pregnant woman, but there are reports alleging six fetal deaths subsequent to use of TASER ECDs, including the one included in the medical literature (Berstein, 1991; DiFilippo, 2012; Heisig, 2011; Ihejirika, 2012; Maddux, 2012; Oakes, 2002).

The single case reported in the medical literature describes a spontaneous abortion in a female heroin user. When she was taken into custody she tested positive for heroin. At the time of the ECD application, she was eight to ten weeks pregnant (Mehl, 1992). While in jail, officers used a the ECD and hit her in the abdomen and the leg. She began spontaneously to miscarry seven days later and received a dilatation and curettage procedure 14 days later for incomplete abortion (Mehl, 1992). No conclusive link with the TASER ECD was proven (Bleetman, Steyn, and Lee, 2004).

Einarson, Bailey, Inocencion, Ormond, and Koren (1997) conducted a study of 31 women who had been exposed to electrical current at various voltage levels during pregnancy. Compared to a control group of 30 women, there were no differences between the groups in pregnancy outcome, birth weight, gestational age, type of delivery, or rates of neonatal distress. The researchers concluded that, in most cases, accidental electric shock occurring during day-to-day life during pregnancy does not pose a major fetal risk. However, none of the women received a shock from a TASER ECD. According to Mehl (1992), the uterus and amniotic fluid are excellent conductors of electric current, so one possible explanation for TASER ECD related fetal death could be cardiac arrest caused by current reaching the fetus. There are no medical studies testing his hypothesis, and none of the studies on TASER ECD-proximate deaths or arrest-related deaths discusses pregnancy.

CHAPTER 3

What We Know About TASER Technology

The debate over potential adverse cardiac effects of TASER ECDs is complex, unsettled, and confounded by the lack of sufficient scientific evidence to reach conclusions under the unusual psychological, physiological, metabolic, and physical conditions of real world applications. There are many limitations to current studies based on epidemiologic observations and clinical studies in healthy volunteers. Important confounding clinical variables, such as ExDS, restraint techniques, presence of underlying cardiovascular disease, metabolic derangements, and the influence of alcohol, stimulants, or other drugs, cannot be controlled in retrospective reviews or reproduced in clinical investigations (Link and Estes, 2008).

CARDIAC EFFECTS OF TASER ECDs

It is well documented in medical literature that external high voltage stimulation of the heart can influence the internal electrical activity of the heart and can lead to cardiac arrhythmia and VF. The effect of the electricity depends on the heart's state of agitation and the current applied. The threshold for the current and voltage required to induce myocardial contractions varies with impulse duration, which means that shorter pulse durations require larger amounts of current to depolarize the cardiac membrane and alter the cardiac rhythm (Kunz, Grove, and Fischer, 2012). This knowledge led to early studies of the cardiac effects of TASER discharges following reports of sudden unexpected deaths.

TASER International funded many of the early studies due to their obvious interest in the results. The results of those studies, which showed no cardiac effect in humans, have been criticized. Azadani, Tseng, Ermakov, Marcus, and Lee (2011) compared the conclusions of studies that were sponsored or funded by TASER International to the conclusions of independently funded studies. They found that studies funded by TASER International and/or written by an author affiliated with the company were substantially more likely to conclude that TASERs were safe, and, thus, research supported by TASER International might be significantly biased in favor of TASER safety.

Many factors promote the argument for TASER ECD safety. First, modeling studies suggest that the electric fields ECDs generate within the thorax are too weak to affect myocardial cells. Second, the duration of the electrical pulses is much shorter than the chronaxie, or the optimal stimulus duration, of the heart. Third, anisotropy, the tendency of the electric current to follow the grain of skeletal muscle, diverts current around rather than though the thoracic cavity. Fourth, the lungs and the perpendicular muscle grain of the *pectoralis major* help to shield the *epicardium* (Kroll, 2009). It is possible that abnormal or diseased hearts are more vulnerable to TASER shocks than normal healthy hearts, but there are no studies of the effects of TASER ECDs on such diseased hearts (Tchou, 2007).

The most common cause of death following both high- and low-voltage electrical injuries is ventricular fibrillation (VF), but survivors can suffer many arrhythmias, from premature ventricular contraction to atrial fibrillation (Primavesi, 2009). If ECDs were to cause death by direct cardiac stimulation, the initial post arrest rhythm should be VF, and subjects should collapse within 10 to 15 seconds after ECD discharge. If collapse is delayed, or the initial rhythm is an idioventricular rhythm, such as asystole or pulseless electrical activity (PEA), then electrically induced VF is not the cause of death (Swerdlow, Fishbein, Chaman, Lakkireddy, and Tchou, 2009). Some medical researchers recommend cardiac monitoring for as long as 24 hours after electrical injuries to prevent deaths from delayed arrhythmias, but arrhythmias in patients after electric shock are uncommon and, if present, are usually visible on the first electrocardiogram (ECG) (Primavesi, 2009).

The X26 produces an average current of 1.9 mA, or about one percent of the current needed to cause the heart of the typical adult male to fibrillate. The heart's chronaxie is about 3 ms, or about 30 times as long as the chronaxie of skeletal muscle nerves and the pulse lengths of a TASER ECD. The single-pulse current required to electrocute someone by directly pulsing the most sensitive part of the heartbeat using 3 ms pulses is about 3 amps. Because of the 100 µs pulse of the TASER ECD, which is only a small fraction of the heart's chronaxie, it would hypothetically take a current of 90 amps to initiate VF as compared to the X26 current of 1.9 mA (Kroll, 2007).

Animal Model Experiments
Scientists often use animals, particularly pigs, as a substitute for humans in medical experiments. Jauchem (2010) cites several reasons why a swine model is appropriate for TASER technology experiments:

- the comparability of domestic pig skin to human skin;
- the similarities of pigs to humans in chemical and physical characteristics of blood, respiratory parameters, and responses to muscular exercise;
- the anatomical and physiological similarity of pigs' lungs to those of humans;
- the equivalence of the ratio of heart size to body weight in pigs and humans;
- the resemblance of coronary arterial distribution of pigs to humans; and
- normal swine intra-cardiac electrophysiological parameters resemble those of humans more closely than any non-primate animal.

However, there are important confounders in swine experiments, including anatomical and electrophysiological differences between humans and pigs, the use of anesthesia, controlled laboratory conditions, and repetitive shocks in animals smaller than humans (Pippin, 2007). Researchers have known since 1936 that swine are unusually sensitive to the electrical induction of VF (Kroll, Panescu, Carver, Kroll, and Hinz, 2009). Pigs provide a conservative model for the risks of the induction of VF, requiring 35 percent less current for the same body mass to induce VF (Kroll, Luceri, and Calkins, 2007). In pigs, the Purkinje fibers that innervate cardiac muscle cross the entire ventricular wall, whereas in dogs and humans they are confined to a thin endocardial layer. Activation of contractions in swine proceeds from the epicardium to the endocardium, whereas it occurs in the reverse direction in dogs and humans. Radiofrequency ablation, routinely done in humans, typically produces VF in swine because they are more sensitive to higher frequencies than are humans (Kroll, Calkins, Luceri, Graham, and Heegaard, 2008).

Despite the fact that pigs are more sensitive than are humans to electrical currents, it is appropriate to use them for relative within-species comparisons. For example, it is scientifically valid to use pigs to study the differential effects of cocaine versus no cocaine or to study the effects of varying body weight on TASER ECD safety margins (Kroll, Panescu, Carver, Kroll, and Hinz, 2009).

Although most TASER technology experiments on animals involve swine models, there are two notable experiments involving cardiac effects on dogs. McDaniel, Stratbucker, and Smith (2000) administered 236 shocks from a first generation TASER ECD to five anesthetized dogs through probes they placed in and on the thorax to maximize the potential for adverse cardiac interactions. The discharges resulted in no episodes of VF. However, in one animal, the researchers could intermittently pace the heart when both TASER probes were directly over the heart. They concluded that the risk of inducing VF in healthy humans by the normal use of early model TASER ECDs was very small.

McDaniel and Stratbucker (2006) anesthetized five dogs and subjected them to shocks from an M26. They placed the probes on the thorax, keeping the heart between the probes to create a worst-case scenario. Four dogs received intravenous epinephrine to increase the heart rate and simulate flight, and three dogs were shocked simultaneously with two devices. The researchers applied 192 discharges from the M26, but they observed no evidence of VF.

Experiments on swine models have tested the effects of TASER technology on cardiac safety by varying, singularly or in combination, current strength, current duration, probe location, number of discharges, and infusion of cocaine. In an experiment with 13 anesthetized adult pigs, Stratbucker, Roeder, and Nerheim (2003) applied 71 discharges of a standard X26 directly into the chests of the animals, configuring the electrodes to maximize the likelihood of cardiac interaction. Standard X26 discharges never produced VF, and the stimulation was insufficient to evoke even an occasional paced beat, which is a much lower stimulus threshold than induction of VF. The researchers increased the intensity of the pulses, but they did not induce VF until they had increased the intensity by 2,000 percent, or 20 times greater than the standard charge.

Another team of researchers conducted a study to compare the standard X26 discharge with the discharge necessary to initiate VF in nine pigs. They anesthetized the animals and continuously monitored their arterial blood pressure, blood oxygen saturation, respiration, and heart rate. They positioned the probes to ensure that the charge was delivered across the thorax. They first applied the standard TASER charge to the animal, increasing the charge with each subsequent application until they induced VF. They found that, directly proportional to the weight of the animal, a discharge 15 to 42 times the standard discharge of the X26 was necessary to induce VF (McDaniel, Stratbucker, Nerheim, and Brewer, 2005).

Lakkireddy, Wallick, Ryschon, Chung, Butany, Martin, Saliba, Kowalewski, Natale, and Tchou (2006) tested five pigs using a custom designed instrument built to deliver multiples of the standard TASER X26 discharge. They applied the discharges in a step-up and step-down fashion using tethered probes at five locations. They observed that a single standard application did not induce VF at any of the five locations.

DeMonte, Wang, Ma, Gao, and Joy (2009) used current density imaging to measure average current density magnitude in the torso of an in-vivo piglet for applied current pulse amplitudes ranging from ten mA to 110 mA. They found that they could apply current pulses exceeding 500 microcoulombs (μC) to the chest of a small piglet near the heart without fatally disrupting cardiac function under the condition that the pulses were applied within a window of about 180 ms following the R-wave of the cardiac cycle. They also noted that other experiments have shown that cardiac function can be disrupted by current pulses with a charge as low as 190 μC when these pulses are applied following the T-wave of the cardiac cycle, but the average output of an X26 is only 80 μC.

Beason, Jauchem, Clark, Parker, and Fines (2009) anesthetized ten pigs and subjected them to pulse waveforms similar to the X26 to test the relative effects of pulse variations on muscle contraction and the possibility of cardiac effects. They found that to reach a 50 percent probability of inducing VF, it would take four to five times more current than a standard X26 discharge. Large variations about the X26 operating level did not result in VF or asystole.

Walcott, Kroll, and Ideker (2011) experimented with five pigs to study the VF risks of a train of multiple short pulses such as those used in a TASER ECD. They placed an electrode through the anterior chest so the tip was ten mm from the *epicardium*, and they attached a return electrode to the lower abdomen. They delivered five-second trains of 100 µs pulses at rates of 10 – 70 PPS with gradually increasing charges until they induced VF. As expected, the VF charge threshold decreased with increasing rates. They concluded that the output of TASER ECDs were well below the VF risk limits in international standards.

Nanthakumar, Billingsley, Massé, Dorian, Cameron, Chauhan, Downar, and Sevaptsidis (2006) noticed that previous studies used only surface ECG monitoring. Electromagnetic interference of the discharge prevented examining the immediate cardiac electrophysiological consequences of the pulse, so they introduced intra-cardiac catheters and blood pressure transducers into six pigs. They tested the M26 and X26 models by applying charges in two vectors: a thoracic vector that ran parallel to the long axis of the heart on the chest wall, and a non-thoracic vector that ran away from the heart across the abdomen. They also investigated two different lengths of discharge, five seconds and 15 seconds. The researchers studied the effects of 150 discharges of a standard TASER ECD. Of those, 94 were thoracic discharges and 56 were non-thoracic.

During the non-thoracic discharges, the researchers observed no stimulation of the *myocardium*. However, they did observe myocardial stimulation in 74 percent of the thoracic discharges. The X26 model was more likely to stimulate the *myocardium* than the M26 model, and the 15-second duration was more likely to stimulate the *myocardium* than the five-second discharge. However, none of the discharges resulted in VT or VF. To simulate conditions of ExDS, they infused the pigs with epinephrine and applied 16 discharges in the thoracic vector. Thirteen of those discharges resulted in stimulation of the *myocardium*. Of those 13 discharges, one resulted in VF and one resulted in non-sustained VT, which spontaneously terminated.

Walter, Dennis, Valentino, Margeta, Nagy, Bokhari, Wiley, Joseph, and Roberts (2008) anesthetized and paralyzed 13 pigs then exposed them to two 40-second discharges from an X26 across the torso. Pre-exposure and at five, 15, 30, and 60 minutes and at 24, 48, and 72 hours post-discharge, they recorded blood pressure, vital signs, blood gases, electrolyte levels, and troponin I (a protein released into the blood by damaged heart muscle). They also performed ECGs and echocardiography before, during, and after the discharges. The ECGs were unreadable during the discharges due to electrical interference, but that interference did not affect echocardiography images. The researchers observed during the discharges, cardiac rhythm was captured immediately at a rate of approximately 300 beats per minute (BPM) in all animals. The capture continued for the duration of the discharge. In three cases, sinus rhythm returned within five seconds of discontinuing the discharge. In two other animals, they observed VF after the discharge by both ECG and echocardiography. In one of those animals, spontaneous reversion to sinus rhythm occurred after 15 seconds, but the other VF resulted in death. Another animal showed VT for fewer than five seconds before reverting to sinus rhythm. In the last three cases, the rhythm during discharge did not change when the discharge ceased. The researchers noted that blood chemistry values were not significantly affected in the post-discharge period. In surviving animals, heart rate was not significantly affected and hypotension was absent.

In an unpublished study from the Institute of Non-Lethal Defense Technologies at The Pennsylvania State University, researchers examined the effects of long-term continuous application of the X26 waveform on anesthetized pigs. In phase one of the study, two pigs, which had not been ventilated, died following less than three minutes of exposure. Researchers observed no indications of breathing or respiratory gas exchange during that time. Noting that research on conscious humans indicated no interruption in breathing, the researchers decided mechanically to ventilate the pigs in the next phase. In phase two, one pig was subjected to a three-minute exposure from an X26, and one pig was subjected to a six-minute exposure. Both pigs survived. In phase three, researchers exposed ten pigs to various exposures from ten to 30 minutes. Two pigs died after about four minutes of exposure, and one pig died after approximately ten minutes. Three of five pigs exposed for 30 minutes survived. The researchers concluded that anesthetized swine would not experience a fatal event when exposed to an X26 for up to three continuous minutes if provided with ventilation, and that there was no dose effect of exposure—the longer applications did not correlate to increased risk of death. They also concluded that their data indicated that metabolic acidosis and cardiac arrhythmias were not likely causes of death (Hughes, Kennett, Murray, Werner, and Jenkins, 2007).

Valentino, Walter, Dennis, Margeta, Starr, Nagy, Bokhari, Wiley, Joseph, and Roberts (2008) anesthetized four pigs, paralyzed them, and exposed them to ten-second discharges from a standard X26. The researchers pushed the probes into the skin to full depth and arranged them in transcardiac and non-transcardiac vectors. They studied 11 different vectors and 22 different discharge conditions, performing echocardiography and ECGs before, during, and after discharge. Although ECGs were not readable during discharge because of electrical interference, echocardiography images demonstrated ventricular rhythm capture in 31 of 59 discharges on the ventral surface. Ventricular capture occurred in 23 of 27 transcardiac vector discharges. The researchers observed ventricular capture in only eight of 32 non-transcardiac discharges. They also observed two instances of VF, both in the transcardiac vector. They concluded that cardiac capture was statistically less likely in the non-transcardiac vectors.

Park, Choi, Ahn, and Min (2013) anesthetized 14 pigs and exposed them to either a five-second or a ten-second discharge. Blood pressure and total peripheral resistance decreased significantly after ECD discharge and returned to baseline values at 15 minutes following the five-second discharges, but they did not return to baseline values during the 30-minute observation period after the ten-second discharges. The researchers concluded that repetitive X26 discharges resulted in adverse cardiovascular events with a dose-response relationship related to the duration of X26 discharges in an anesthetized swine model.

Lakkireddy, Kowalski, Wallick, Verma, Martin, Ryschon, Butany, Natale, and Tchou (2006) anesthetized 13 adult pigs and applied TASER discharges at increasing multiples of standard output in five paired-probe positions until they induced VF. The researchers found that fibrillation thresholds were lowest when they applied the probes in the axis of the heart with one probe at the sternal notch. They observed the highest values when they applied the pulses furthest away from the heart. They noted that, even in the worst-case scenario with the probes plunged fully toward the heart, they were never able to induce VF using a standard discharge.

Tchou, Lakkireddy, and Wallick (2007) positioned X26 probes in five configurations on the torsos of 13 anesthetized pigs. They observed that the current output equivalent to a standard X26 discharge did not induce VF in any pig in any of the five configurations.

Webster, Will, Sun, Wu, O'Rourke, Huebner, and Rahko (2006) anesthetized ten pigs and placed the probes of an X26 in various locations to determine the probe-to-heart distance necessary to induce

VF. The mean probe-to-heart distance that caused VF was 17 mm (± 6.48 mm) for the first VF event and 13.7 mm (± 6.79 mm) for the average of successive VF events in the same location. The researchers concluded that when the probe is close enough to the heart, the current from an X26 could directly trigger VF in pigs. They also noted that echocardiography of erect humans revealed skin-to-heart distances from ten to 57 mm.

Wu, Sun, O'Rourke, Huebner, Rahko, Will, and Webster (2008) noted that in the previous study immediately above researchers had placed the TASER probe into a bluntly dissected pathway that they had filled with a conductive gel to exclude air. The gel unintentionally permitted a more direct electrical pathway to the heart that likely increased the probe-to-heart distance where the TASER ECD could cause VF. In this experiment, the researchers positioned a blunt probe through surrounding tissues without the conductive gel. The mean probe-to-heart distance that caused VF was 6.2 mm (± 1.79 mm) for the first VF event and 5.4 mm (± 2.41 mm) for the average of successive VF events in the same location. The researchers concluded that the reduction in the probe-to-heart distance clearly indicated that the previous procedure using conductive gel substantially increased the distance at which the ECD could induce VF, presumably by reducing the resistance of the pathway from probe to heart.

Lakkireddy, Wallick, Verma, Ryschon, Kowaleski, Wazni, Butany, Martin, and Tchou (2008) attached X26 probes at either the sternal notch or the point of maximum impulse and moved the second probe towards the other at distance intervals of approximately 2.5 centimeters (cm) along the axis on seven pigs. They studied ventricular capture at one standard application. The researchers concluded that myocardial capture ratio decreased with increasing probe separation up to 15 cm in the cardiac axis. However, even in the closest possible application along the cardiac axis, TASER current application induced no VF.

Experimental data have established that an electrode will capture the heart with a significantly lower charge when the electrode touching the cardiac tissue is a cathode. Experimental data also show that there is no difference in the ability of the anode versus the cathode to induce VF. Consequently, Kroll, Panescu, Carver, Kroll, and Hinz (2009) evaluated the effect of polarity changes on cardiac capture and the induction of VF regarding the X26. They anesthetized and ventilated a small swine, located the apex of the heart via echocardiography, and fully inserted TASER probes towards the apex. They used echocardiography to monitor cardiac contractions to determine cardiac capture. They delivered charges of the standard X26, which is 100 µC, and charges of 72 µC to 375 µC at 19 PPS for 15 seconds to test for cardiac capture. There was no cardiac capture with the metered 72 µC charge, but the results were different with the X26. The TASER ECD created cardiac capture, but not VF, 16 out of 21 applications. There was no difference between the cathode or anode capture rates. There was no induction of VF at pulse charges up to 300 µC, and the difference in VF induction rates of pulse charges of 340 – 375 µC for cathode stimulation versus anode stimulation was not significant.

Scientists have long recognized two methods of inducing VF with electrical currents: (1) delivering a brief high-charged shock during the cardiac T-wave, and (2) delivering lower level currents for one to five seconds. However, Kroll, Panescu, Hinz, and Lakkireddy (2010) tested a theoretical third mechanism, which requires delivering current suffi-cient to cause high-rate cardiac capture. Cardiac capture causes cardiac output collapse. If the output collapse is sufficiently long, it leads to ischemia, which, in turn, lowers the VF threshold to the level of the current, which, finally, results in VF. This process requires approxi-mately 40 percent of the normal VF induction current, but it requires minutes instead of seconds to induce VF. They anesthetized and venti-lated six pigs then delivered from a probe tip ten mm from the *epicardium* an electric current that was sufficient to cause hypotensive capture but not sufficient to induce VF within five seconds. After about 90 seconds, on average, VF was induced. The authors noted that this third mechanism of inducing VF could have safety implications relevant to long-term exposures from TASER ECDs and warranted further studies.

Following concerns that intoxication from methamphetamine created greater risks for people exposed to shock from a TASER ECD, Dawes, Ho, Cole, Reardon, Lundin, Terwey, Falvey, and Miner (2010) infused 16 Dorset sheep with methamphetamine. They recorded the sheep's cardiac rhythms and took arterial blood samples at baseline and at each experimental intervention. They gave each sheep 0.0, 0.5, 1.0, or 1.5 mg of methamphetamine per kilogram of body weight. All animals then received ECD exposures in sequences of five, 15, 30, and 40 seconds with a three-minute rest between applications. The researchers observed that all the animals demonstrated signs of methamphetamine intoxication, including atrial and ventricular ectopy, before exposure. The smaller animals exhibited supraventricular arrhythmias and the larger animals exhibited sinus tachycardia after exposures. One of the smaller animals experienced ventricular ectopy, including a run of VT that spontaneously resolved. Five animals of varying size had reliable cardiac capture during exposure but no VF, and they returned to sinus tachycardia when the application stopped.

In the only animal model experiment of the effects of cocaine on TASER technology, Lakkireddy, Wallick, Ryschon, Chung, Butany, Martin, Saliba, Kowalewski, Natale, and Tchou (2006) found that infusion of cocaine into five pigs increased ECD cardiac safety margins by 50 to 100 percent above baseline safety margins, thereby *decreasing* the risk of an adverse cardiac effect.

Computer and Mathematical Studies
Because direct experimentation on the cardiac effects of TASER ECDs on humans is not always possible because of medical limitations and ethical considerations, scientists have turned to computer modeling and mathematical computations to estimate the effects on the heart. Basic calculations derive from the strength-duration formula for current density that can be used to predict the likelihood of induction of VF. The strength-duration formula is:

$$I = I_{Rh} * (1 + c/d)$$

where I is current measured in milliamps per centimeter^2 (mA/cm^2), I_{Rh} is rheobase current measured in mA/cm^2, c is myocyte chronaxie measured in milliseconds (ms), and d is pulse duration measured in microseconds (µs) (Panescu, 2007). The rheobasic current density for long durations required to induce VF in humans is 7 mA/cm^2 (Sun, Wu, Abdallah, and Webster, 2005). For the X26, the current pulse is about 100 µs. The myocyte chronaxie is about 1.2 ms for a human VF model. Consequently, the strength-duration formula is:

$$I = 7 \text{ mA/cm}^2 * (1 + 1.2 \text{ ms/100 µs})$$
$$\text{or}$$
$$I = 91 \text{ mA/cm}^2.$$

Stratbucker, Kroll, McDaniel, and Panescu (2006) found that the estimated maximum current density in the heart volume produced by a standard TASER ECD discharge was 2.7 mA/cm^2, or approximately three percent of the 91 mA/cm^2 current level required to induce VF.

Researchers in England assessed the risk of adverse cardiac events from the M26 and the X26 by modeling the path of current flow in the body using computational electromagnetic modeling. They predicted current flow in the heart and used that data to enable the application of appropriate currents to a biological model—an isolated beating heart preparation called a Langendorff preparation. The researchers could assess the risk of ventricular ectopic beats and VF and then compare that data with other evidence concerning the risks of the TASER ECD to provide an overall medical view on the risks. The researchers programmed the values of current density and waveform shape determined by the modeling study into a simulator for the biological testing phase of the safety study using a Langendorff preparation. The researchers concluded, based on the Langendorff preparation study, that it was unlikely that discharges from the M26 and the X26 could influence cardiac rhythm by direct action on the heart (Defence Science and Technology Laboratory, 2005).

The Joint Non-Lethal Weapons Human Effects Center of Excellence published a report on human effectiveness and risk characterization for TASER ECDs by extrapolating data from animal studies to human thresholds. The researchers could not say what specific anatomical features, such as body fat, skin thickness, distance from the skin surface to the heart, or heart size, were responsible for changes in cardiac effects from the electromagnetic incapacitation charge, so the degree of correlation among those parameters in human populations was not evaluated. Based on the analysis, and assuming that the TASER probe hit the target and established a circuit that crossed the heart, the VF threshold, relative to the X26 output, could be calculated from the dose-response curves for normal persons without potentially sensitizing conditions. Based on threshold estimates, the researchers concluded that, for large children and adults, even those who were sensitive responders, the risk of inducing VF was very small. Consequently, a large safety margin existed. For example, the VF threshold for a 40-pound child was 3.5 times greater than the normal X26 operating output. The threshold for a 200-pound person was 19 times greater than the normal operating output for the typical person and 11 times greater for a person in sensitive populations (Maier, et al., 2005).

Sun, et al. (2005) constructed a simple axisymmetric finite element method model to calculate and estimate current density around a TASER probe. Knowing the rheobasic current density and time constant necessary to induce VF, they calculated the charge density of the M26 and the X26. Thus, they could calculate the current density at any location on the body for any current value inserted into the TASER probe. They determined that the minimum probe-to-heart distances required to induce VF in humans was 7 mm for the X26 and 6 mm for the M26.

Kroll, Sweeney, and Swerdlow (2006) calculated theoretical safety thresholds of new generation TASER ECDs. The minimum current for stimulating A-ά motor neurons is approximately one amp with a chronaxie of 100 μs. For cardiac stimulus at one amp, the chronaxie is three to five ms for transcutaneous stimulation, which is 50 times longer than the standard TASER pulse. Because the heart is located deep within the torso, transcutaneous pulses delivered through large antero-posterior electrodes for optimal cardiac stimulation, such as an external defibrillator, deliver only four percent of their current through the heart. An X26 delivers a much smaller fraction through small probe electrodes used for skeletal muscular incapacitation when positioned on the same side of the abdomen, thorax, or lower extremities. Mathematical computations of the strength-duration relationship demonstrate that the 100 μs pulse length of the TASER pseudo-monophasic waveform is insufficient to pace the heart by a 3:1 safety margin, even if the charge is delivered through large electrodes optimally placed for cardiac stimulation.

The ratio between the current required to pace the heart and that required to induce fatal VF depends on the duration of stimulation and pulse repetition rate; in published animal studies the ratio is between four and six to one, meaning it takes four to six times more current to cause VF than is required to pace the heart. Combining the theoretical 3:1 safety margin from the strength-duration analysis with an average 5:1 estimate for the pacing-to-fibrillation threshold produces a theoretical estimate of a 15:1 safety margin, even if X26 pulses are delivered through electrodes optimized for cardiac stimulation.

Electroporation, an opening of pores in cellular membranes caused by electrical stimulation, results in damage to tissue and increases the conductivity of that tissue, an effect which could decrease the safety thresholds of TASER ECDs. Constructing worst-case assumptions for TASER electrode penetration and separation, Panescu, Kroll, Efimov, and Sweeney (2006) used computer modeling to analyze skeletal muscle and motor nerve activation, cell electroporation, and current and electric field distributions through skin, fat and muscle layers. The analysis predicted worst-case current density and field-strength values higher than thresholds required for neuromuscular activation, but significantly lower than levels needed for permanent cellular electroporation or tissue damage.

Stratbucker, et al. (2006) analyzed strength-duration thresholds for myocyte excitation and VF induction with worst-case TASER electrode placement. The models predicted maximum TASER current density of 0.27 mA/cm^2 in the heart. The researchers determined that numerically simulated heart current density was about half the threshold for myocyte excitation and more than 500 times the current was required to induce VF.

Combining data from swine model studies on probe-to-heart distances and data on TASER probe location studies, Webster, et al. (2006) calculated the probability of a TASER ECD directly triggering VF. They concluded that the probability of a probe landing on the body within one cm^2 over the ventricle and causing VF was about 0.000172, or 172 per 1,000,000 applications.

Holden, Sheridan, Coffey, Scaramuzza, and Diamantopoulos (2007) used a numerical phantom constructed from medical images of the human body in which the material properties of the tissues are represented to determine the arrhythmogenic potential of the M26 and X26 waveforms. Computational electromagnetic modeling predicted the currents arising at the heart following application of the waveforms at the anterior surface of the chest with one TASER probe directly overlying the ventricles. The modeling indicated that the peak absolute current densities at the ventricles were 0.66 mA/mm^2 for the M26 waveform and 0.11 mA/mm^2 for the X26 waveform.

During the T-wave, they applied those current densities and waveforms to the ventricular epicardial surface of guinea-pig isolated hearts. They observed no ectopic beats or VF with a standard discharge. The M26 and X26 waveforms induced ectopic beats only at current densities greater than 60-fold those predicted by the computer modeling. When applied to the ventricles in trains designed to mimic the discharge patterns of ECDs, neither waveform induced VF at peak currents. Currents greater than 70-fold for the M26 waveform and greater than 240-fold for the X26 waveform were needed to induce VF.

Sun (2007) estimated the VF probability and motor nerve stimulation caused by an X26 given data from swine probe-to-heart studies, minimum human skin-to-heart distances, and field use probe landing statistics. The estimated mean of the probability of human VF was 0.0008, or eight in 10,000, using resected (surgically removed) chest wall swine study data and 0.000015, or 15 in 1,000,000, using blunt probe swine study data. The dangerous radius had a mean of 7.9 mm with a maximum of 53.2 mm indicating that the probe landing in a small frontal region over the heart was a necessary, but not sufficient, condition for the X26 to induce VF.

Panescu (2007) estimated the current flow and effects of M26 and X26 waveform discharges on the human body. Energy values for muscle regions were significantly higher than neuromuscular activation thresholds. Even with an unrealistically thin layer of fat and worst-case skeletal muscle, maximum values for current densities and electric field strengths were lower, by at least a factor of seven, than levels reported to produce permanent cellular electroporation or tissue damage. Even with an unrealistically thin layer of fat and worst-case skeletal muscle, maximum values for current densities that reach into deeper layers of tissue were insufficient to trigger VF.

Using the fundamental law of electrostimulation and experimental data from the available literature, Ideker and Dosdall (2007) calculated the likelihood that the X26 could induce VF either immediately or sometime after its use. The researchers reasoned that, because of the short duration of TASER pulses, the long chronaxie of cardiac cells, the small fraction of current from electrodes on the body surface that passes through the heart, and the resultant high pacing threshold from the body surface, the fundamental law of electrostimulation predicted that TASER pulses would not stimulate an ectopic beat in the large majority of normal adults. They argued since the immediate initiation of VF in a normal heart requires a very premature stimulated ectopic beat and the threshold for such premature beats is higher than less premature beats it was unlikely that TASER pulses could immediately initiate VF in such individuals through the direct effect of the electric field generated through the heart by the TASER ECD. In the absence of preexisting heart disease, the delayed development of VF required the electrical stimuli to cause electroporation or myocardial necrosis.

However, the electrical thresholds for electroporation and necrosis are many times higher than that required to stimulate an ectopic beat. Therefore, they concluded, it is highly unlikely that the X26 could cause VF minutes to hours after its use through direct cardiac effects of the electric field.

Panescu, Kroll, and Stratbucker (2008), using finite element models, determined that skin, fat, and anisotropic skeletal muscle layers shunt a large portion of currents allowing just a fraction of the energy to penetrate into deeper layers of tissue. They calculated that the theoretical probability of inducing VF was lower than 0.0000008, or approximately 0.8 per 1,000,000 applications. They noted, for comparison, that international safety standards for electrical medical equipment accept a VF induction probability rate of 0.002, or one per 500 uses.

Panescu, Kroll, and Stratbucker (2009) noted that concerns had been raised about the use of TASER ECDs in 3-point deployment, with two drive-stun electrodes on a suspect's back and a probe electrode lodged into the suspect's chest. They constructed finite element models to approximate current density in the heart for worst-case three-point probe placement. The models analyzed strength-duration thresholds for myocyte excitation and VF induction and estimated that maximum current densities in the heart and in neighboring organs were at safe levels. When they compared a three-point deployment mode to probe mode deployment, the margins of safety for the three-point deployment were estimated to be as high as or higher than the probe-mode deployment. The researchers concluded that their numerical modeling estimated that TASER ECDs in drive-stun, probe-mode, or three-point deployments had high theoretically approximated safety margins for cardiac capture, VF, and skeletal muscle damage by electroporation.

Kroll, Panescu, Brewer, Lakkireddy, and Graham (2009) reviewed eight peer-reviewed papers studying the application of chest exposures from an X26 in which the heart was in the current path between the barbs. These studies reported 117 chest exposures in 81 swine weighing between 22 and 117 kilograms. There were three inductions of VF in 56 swine that weighed fewer than 37 kilograms, but there were no reports of VF in swine weighing more than 37 kilograms. Scaling the weights using classical data ratios, the researchers determined that the maximum human weight at which VF was likely was 13.3 kilograms, or approximately 29.3 pounds (confidence interval

15.6 to 46.6 pounds). They predicted the probability of an X26 causing VF in a human weighing 91 kilograms (200 pounds), which is the mean weight of reported ExDS deaths, to be 0.0000000000034, or 3.4 per 1,000,000,000,000 applications.

Sun, Haemmerich, Rahko, and Webster (2010) estimated the order of probability for TASER ECDs directly causing human VF by using: (1) current densities near the human heart estimated by using 3D finite-element models; (2) prior data of the maximum probe-to-heart distances that caused VF in pigs; (3) minimum skin-to-heart distances measured in erect humans by echocardiography; and (4) probe landing distribution estimated from police reports. They estimated the mean probability of human VF was 0.001(one in 1,000) for data from pigs having a chest wall resected to the ribs and 0.000006 (6 in 1,000,000) for data from a pig with no resection when inserting a blunt probe. The VF probability for a given probe location decreased with the probe-to-heart horizontal distance (radius) on the skin surface. They argued that there was very strong evidence against the hypothesis that VF probability was zero.

Leitgeb, Niedermayr, Loos, and Neubauer (2011) estimated VF risk of TASER pulses based on sophisticated numerical modeling of cardiac cells and human anatomy, which allowed studying myocardial reaction to short TASER pulses. They argued that the overall risk was very low, but that it was implausible that the risk was as low as the 0.0000008 (0.8 in 1,000,000) risk that Panescu, et al. (2009) had estimated. Due to the small risk and its dependence on various additional factors such as positioning of the electrodes and individual anatomy, they argued that experiments with such small numbers could not lead to consistent results.

Human Model Experiments
Although animal studies have produced evidence of potentially fatal cardiac effects in pigs, no human model experiment has produced evidence of VT or VF. In only one experiment did researchers observe evidence of potential cardiac capture. That experiment was conducted with a new model ECD that was under development but not yet in production (Ho, Dawes, Reardon, Strote, Kunz, Nelson, Lundin, Orozco, and Miner, 2011). Some researchers, however, have criticized human experiments for not reflecting real world conditions (Strote and Hutson, 2009).

Researchers at the University of California – San Diego conducted a series of four experiments on law enforcement officers undergoing training on the use of TASER ECDs. The first experiment was a prospective pilot study to evaluate cardiac changes using three-lead ECG monitoring immediately before, during, and after application of an X26. The researchers collected data on 20 volunteer subjects. The mean shock duration was 2.4 seconds, with a range of 1.2 to five seconds. Other than sinus tachycardia, the researchers observed no arrhythmias. There was no change in morphology, QRS duration, or QT interval between the before and after data, although there was a decrease in the PR interval. The mean heart rate increased 15 BPM. The researchers concluded in this pilot study that there were no significant cardiac arrhythmias in healthy subjects immediately after receiving an X26 discharge (Levine, Sloane, Chan, Vilke, and Dunford, 2005).

The second study was a prospective study again performed with law enforcement officers receiving training on the X26. The officers had continuous ECG monitoring immediately before, during, and after the application of the X26 to determine changes in cardiac rate, rhythm, and morphology. The researchers enrolled 76 subjects, nine of whom they later excluded because of equipment malfunction. For the remaining 67 subjects, the mean shock duration was 2.2 seconds, with a range of 0.9 to five seconds. The researchers found that the mean heartbeat increased 19.4 BPM, but they observed no significant changes in the QRS morphology or any aberrant beats. They did find one subject who had a single premature ventricular contraction before and after the TASER shock, but no other subject had any other arrhythmia except sinus tachycardia (Levine, Sloane, Chan, Vilke, and Dunford, 2006a).

In the third study, the researchers enrolled 58 law enforcement officers who were receiving training on the use of the X26. Researchers later excluded nine subjects because of ECG lead displacement during the application. In the remaining 49 subjects, the mean shock duration was 2.3 seconds, with a range of 1.2 to five seconds. The subjects displayed an increase in mean heart rate of 20 BPM, but there were no significant changes in PR, QRS, or QT intervals. One subject had rare unifocal premature ventricular contractions pre- and post-discharge, but the researchers found no other arrhythmias except sinus tachycardia (Levine, Sloane, Chan, Vilke, and Dunford, 2006b).

In the fourth experiment, researchers enrolled 115 law enforcement officers in training on the use of the X26. They later excluded 10 subjects due to ECG leads becoming dislodged during the application. The average shock duration was three seconds, with a range of 0.9 to five seconds. The study included evaluation of cardiac rate, rhythm, morphology, interval duration, and the presence of ectopic beats. Four researchers independently conducted blinded analyses of the tracings. They found a significant increase in heart rate, but they identified no cardiac rhythm disturbances or morphologies except for a few subjects who appeared to have prolonged QT changes, the significance of which was unclear (Levine, Sloane, Chan, Dunford, and Vilke, 2007).

Barnes, Winslow, Alson, Johnson, and Bozeman (2006) sought to determine cardiac rhythm effects from TASER ECD exposure and to evaluate those effects for potential dose response relationships, including change in heart rate, rhythm, and morphology. Twenty-nine police officers, who were participating in training and testing, underwent one-second, three-second, and five-second exposures with continuous ECG monitoring before, during, and after exposure. The researchers measured blood pressure at rest before and approximately one minute after exposure. They analyzed ECGs to determine heart rate, rhythm, and morphology using statistical analysis to evaluate differences in the measured parameters. They observed normal sinus rhythm or sinus tachycardia before and after each exposure, but they observed no cardiac arrhythmias. The electrical interference that the ECD produced usually obscured cardiac rhythms during exposure, but researchers were able to discern an underlying sinus rhythm in some cases. Although the shocks produced statistically significant increases in heart rate, they produced no arrhythmias, and researchers observed no dose response relationship.

Ho, Luceri, Lakkireddy, and Dawes (2006) examined whether human exposure to a standard TASER ECD caused detectable changes in 12-lead ECGs. The researchers enrolled 32 volunteer subjects to undergo a five-second application with deployed probes from approximately seven feet using a standard X26. The researchers performed serial ECGs on all subjects immediately before and immediately after TASER exposure, and again at 16 and 24 hours after exposure. A blinded cardiologist interpreted the ECGs. At baseline, 30 of the 32 ECGs were normal. The two abnormal ECGs remained unchanged at all four evaluations. The researchers noted no other ECG abnormalities and detected no changes from baseline.

Barnes, Winslow, Johnson, Alson, Phillips, and Bozeman (2007) enrolled 28 volunteers to undergo one-second, three-second, and five-second exposures to an X26 while performing continuous ECG monitoring before, during, and after each exposure. They analyzed the ECGs to determine heart rate, rhythm, and morphology, and they measured blood pressure at rest before and approximately one minute after the initial exposure. They recorded normal sinus rhythm or sinus tachycardia before and after each exposure, but they observed no cardiac arrhythmias. Mean heart rate increased in each test group, and heart rate tended to increase with longer duration of TASER exposure. Mean blood pressure increased after the standard five-second X26 discharge. The researchers observed that the TASER shocks did produce a statistically significant increase in heart rate, but they observed no detectable arrhythmias and no dose response relationship.

Vilke, Sloane, Bouton, Kolkhorst, Levine, Neuman, Castillo, and Chan (2007) took baseline cardiovascular measurements and blood samples from 8 volunteers. The test subjects then exercised to 85 percent of maximum heart rate. Researchers took a second set of blood samples when subjects reached the predicted heart rate. The subjects then received a five-second TASER ECD exposure. The researchers rechecked blood samples at one, 10, 30, and 60 minutes post-discharge. They measured cardiovascular markers, including systolic and diastolic blood pressures and heart rate, at five, 15, 30, 45, and 60 minutes post-exposure. From a slightly elevated baseline prior to exposure, systolic blood pressure and heart rate decreased linearly post-exercise through the observation period. Oxygen levels never dropped below 96 percent for any measure interval. The researchers noted that no changes were clinically significant.

Vilke, Sloane, Levine, Neuman, Castillo, and Chan (2008) monitored 32 subjects' baseline 12-lead ECGs immediately before and within one minute after a TASER discharge and examined changes in cardiac rhythm, morphology, and interval duration. All subjects had an interpretable 12-lead ECG obtained before and after the TASER ECD activation, although one subject's post-exposure pulse rate interval could not be determined. There were significant changes in heart rate, pulse rate interval, and QT interval among subjects with a normal body mass index, and in pulse rate interval among those who were overweight or obese. However, the researchers noted that none of the statistically significant differences between ECG measures was clinically relevant.

Bozeman, Barnes, Winslow, Johnson, Phillips, and Alson (2009) enrolled 28 volunteer police officers who were participating in TASER ECD training to undergo one-second, three-second, or five-second discharges. The researchers continuously monitored ECGs before, during, and after each of 84 exposures. They also measured blood pressures at rest before and within one minute of exposure. ECD exposure produced no detectable arrhythmias, although it did produce a statistically significant increase in heart rate.

VanMeenen, Cherniack, Bergen, Gleason, Teichman, and Servatius (2010) conducted experiments with 118 law enforcement trainees who received shocks from an X26 for up to 5 seconds. Of the participants, 109 received the full five-second application, one received a four-second discharge, six received three seconds, and two received two seconds. They also varied the method of transmission: 66 participants received the discharge through probes, and 52 received the discharge through alligator clips applied to clothing. Although the location varied, all exposures took place on the back of the body. The researchers observed no evidence of cardiac or skeletal muscle breakdown. Exposure did not adversely affect ECG morphology obtained 24 hours after exposure in 99 trainees. For two trainees with preexisting ECG abnormalities, ECG morphology differed in the post-ECD samples. Ninety-two participants had normal ECG recordings pre- and post-exposure and 9 participants showed ECG abnormalities pre- and post-exposure. The average PR interval, QRS interval, QT interval, and axis deviations had no significant mean changes 24 hours after exposure. Additionally, there was no evidence of cardiac cell death, and troponin I was undetectable, or less than 0.1 nanogram per milliliter (ng/mL). Exposure to the X26 did not affect cardiac and muscle enzymes or measures on the metabolic panel.

Ho, Dawes, Heegaard, Calkins, Moscati, and Miner (2011) obtained baseline ECGs from 25 volunteers then put those volunteers through a regimen of timed push-ups and a sprint on a treadmill until subjective exhaustion to simulate the physical exertion often seen in subjects prior to ECD application in the field. The volunteers then received a continuous 15-second application from an X26 at random positions of the electrodes on their thoraces, either both electrodes in front or both in back. Electrode positions involved at least a 12-inch spread and always encompassed the normal anatomic position of the heart. Following the exposure, researchers obtained an ECG that was interpreted by a blinded cardiologist. The researchers found that, at baseline, 24 of the 25 ECGs were normal. One baseline ECG was abnormal due to several monomorphic premature ventricular complexes. The cardiologist interpreted all 25 ECGs as normal.

Research had demonstrated that the application of a TASER ECD could cause cardiac capture in pigs, but no one had observed the phenomenon in humans. Ho, Reardon, Dawes, Johnson, and Miner (2007) opined that exposures due to artifact interference between the ECD probe and the ECG electrodes prevented researchers from observing cardiac effects during the discharge in humans and could obscure real-time cardiac effects, so they examined real-time cardiac rate measurement using cardiac ultrasound technology. Thirty-seven adult volunteers underwent echocardiography before and after an anaerobic exertion regimen immediately followed by a 15-second exposure with pre-placed thoracic electrodes. They also performed limited real-time echocardiography during the application. An emergency physician trained in ultrasonography analyzed the images for evidence of tachyarrhythmia and observed no adverse events. The mean heart rate prior to starting the event increased immediately following exercise. During exposure the mean heart rate increased slightly, but it dropped one minute after exposure. Sinus rhythm was clearly demonstrated in 18 subjects during exposure, but sinus rhythm was not clearly demonstrated in 19 subjects due to movement artifact. However, heart rate was never greater than 156 BPM in any of the subjects.

Dawes, Ho, Reardon, and Miner (2010) deployed TASER probes from seven feet into the chests of ten volunteer human subjects. They had modified the ECD to discharge the probes but not to deliver a shock. After they had positioned the volunteer, they connected the original cartridge to a standard X26 and subjected each volunteer to a standard five-second discharge. A physician expert in ultrasonography examined an electrocardiographic view to determine heart rhythm before, during, and after the discharge. One subject moved during the application, so the result for that one volunteer was inconclusive. For the other nine volunteers, the researchers observed normal sinus rhythm, and there was no evidence of cardiac capture.

Ho, Dawes, Reardon, Lapine, Dolan, Lundin, and Miner (2008) enrolled 34 volunteer subjects to undergo limited echocardiography before, during, and after a ten-second application of an X26 with preplaced electrodes in the upper right sternal border and the cardiac apex. Sinus rhythm was clearly demonstrated in 21 subjects during exposure. Rhythm was not clearly demonstrated in the other subjects due to artifact movement, but the researchers observed no adverse cardiac events.

Ho, Dawes, Reardon, Lapine, Olsen, Lundin, and Miner (2008) enrolled 44 adult volunteer subjects to undergo limited echo-cardiography before, during and after a 15-second application from an X26 with pre-placed electrodes. Researchers placed the electrodes in a cardiac axis position at the upper left or right sternal border and the estimated cardiac apex. An emergency physician trained in ultra-sonography analyzed the images for evidence of arrhythmia. The mean heart rate prior to starting the event was 105.6 BPM. During exposure, the mean heart rate was 123.3 BPM decreasing to 93.9 BPM one minute after exposure. Researchers clearly observed sinus rhythm in 28 subjects during exposure. They did not clearly observe sinus rhythm in 16 subjects due to movement artifact. They observed no adverse cardiac events, and they were unable to reproduce the tachycardia that other researchers had found in animal models.

Ho, Dawes, Reardon, Moscati, Gardner, and Miner (2008) enrolled 21 law enforcement officers and physicians who were attending training in the use of TASER ECDs to undergo exposures in drive stun mode from an X26. The volunteers received two five-second applications with a one-second rest period between shocks while receiving either limited cardiac or right-hemidiaphragm ultra-sonography. Ten subjects had cardiac views, and 11 had diaphragm views. All applications were delivered either to the trapezius or to lower extremities. The researchers observed that all cardiac rhythms were normal sinus rhythms throughout the observation period.

In a book chapter on the effects of TASER ECDs, Reardon (2009) reported on two previously unpublished studies of echocardiographic monitoring of human subjects during exposures. In the first study, researchers enlisted 12 volunteers to be exposed to a standard five-second exposure. A physician sonographer obtained and interpreted views of the heart in real time during the exposures. In ten volunteers, the cardiac rhythm and gross left ventricular functions were unchanged.

Movement in two subjects made it impossible to obtain echocardiographic images.

In the second study, researchers enlisted the assistance of 60 volunteers and subjected each to a ten-second exposure from an X26. A physician sonographer obtained a view of the heart during exposure and digitally recorded the images for later evaluation. Several blinded cardiologists later read the images. Although the left ventricle was clearly visualized in all cases, the cardiologists' interpretations were inconsistent, even when the same images were shown to the same cardiologists twice. In about 90 percent of the subjects, the left ventricle was judged to be grossly normal. In the other ten percent, the quality of the images was not adequate to judge ventricular function. Nevertheless, in neither study did researchers observe evidence of cardiac capture or tachyarrhythmia.

Ho, Dawes, Reardon, Strote, Kunz, Nelson, Lundin, Orozco, and Miner (2011) enlisted 45 volunteers in training courses to receive a probe deployment to the frontal torso in one of three configurations: two, three, or four embedded probes. The volunteers then experienced a ten-second exposure. Researchers recorded vital signs, ECGs, and serum troponin I values before and after exposure. They also used real-time echocardiography before, during, and after the exposure to evaluate heart rate and rhythm. Initially, they used a version of an ECD that was in the final stages of manufacturer verification that was not yet released. During an exposure with two probes, researchers observed an apparent brief episode of cardiac capture in one subject. They immediately halted testing and notified the manufacturer. The manufacturer redesigned the ECD, and researchers continued the study using the newer version on 45 volunteers. They observed no evidence of cardiac capture and no changes in ECG morphology or troponin I.

Researchers questioned whether the current from a TASER ECD could result in myocardial injury without being observed on ECGs or echocardiography. Sixty-six law enforcement officers receiving training in the use of the X26 volunteered to have a single serum troponin I measured six hours after they received a discharge as part of their training. Troponin I values for all subjects were less than 0.2 ng/mL (a positive assay being defined as greater than 0.2 ng/mL) indicating no myocardial necrosis (Sloane, Vilke, Chan, Levine, and Dunford, 2007; Sloan, Chan, Levine, Dunford, Neuman, and Vilke, 2008).

Ho, Dawes, Cole, and Miner (2008) enlisted four volunteers to experience an exposure to the civilian model TASER ECD, the C2. Three volunteers experienced a 20-second discharge, and one volunteer experienced a 30-second discharge to the thorax. Researchers drew venous blood before, immediately after, and 24 hours post-discharge to analyze biomarkers of acidosis and cellular damage, and they recorded ECGs before and after exposure. They observed no significant changes in ECGs or troponin I levels.

Dawes, Ho, Reardon, Sweeney, and Miner (2010) enrolled 16 volunteers and exposed them to multiple simultaneous five-second discharges to the chest, back, chest-abdomen, and thighs. They analyzed blood samples for troponin I before and 24 hours after discharge. They had a blinded cardiologist interpret ECGs they recorded before and during discharge. They also had a physician, who was an expert in ultrasonography, read echocardiograms in real time during discharge on six of the volunteers. The researchers found that troponin I levels were within normal ranges at all times. ECG changes reflected only increases in vagal tone, which are impulses from the vagus nerve that influence heartbeat. In four of the six subjects who had echocardiograms, the echocardiographer observed normal sinus rhythm during discharge.

Previous studies showed site sensitivity of cardiac capture in pigs depending on the location of the TASER probes and their distance from the heart. Human studies had not demonstrated any induced arrhythmias; however, it was unclear whether previous investigators had placed the electrodes at the most vulnerable regions of the chest. Bashian, Wagner, Wallick, and Tchou (2007) analyzed 45 cardiac computed tomography (CT) scans from randomly selected patients to determine the minimum skin-to-heart distance and the location of that point on the chest surface relative to anatomic landmarks, specifically the horizontal distance from mid sternum and vertical distance from sternal insertion of the lowest left rib. They found that minimum skin-to-heart distances ranged from 1.8 cm to 6.4 cm. The minimum skin-to-heart distance was 2.5 cm to the left of mid sternum and 0.5 cm inferior to the lowest left rib sternal insertion. The area of myocardial contact with the anterior chest wall averaged 51 cm^2 and was unrelated to body mass index. They noted that there was a linear relationship between body mass index and minimum skin-to-heart distances. They concluded that the size of a person and the anatomic relationship of the heart to the anterior chest wall could influence the potential cardiac capture by ECDs at the site of minimum skin-to-heart distance.

Rahko (2008) noted that data from a swine model experiment suggested that a TASER probe placed within 17 mm of the epicardial surface could cause VF (Webster, et al., 2006). He performed two-dimensional echocardiograms in 150 standing adults in three views and measured the shortest linear skin-to-heart distance in each view. He found that six percent of the individuals had a skin-to-heart distance less than or equal to 17 mm. The skin-to-heart distance was significantly correlated with body mass index. He concluded that a TASER probe penetrating the skin directly over the heart might put some individuals at risk for VF.

Swerdlow, Kroll, Williams, Biria, Lakkireddy, and Tchou (2008) requested autopsy records for sudden deaths following the use of TASER ECDs during the period 2001 to 2006. Cases for this study included only incidents wherein the decedent collapsed within 15 minutes of discharge and records indicated a rhythm diagnosis by a physician, paramedic, or automatic external defibrillator (AED). They classified rhythms analyzed by AEDs as "no shock advised" as asystole or PEA. They classified rhythms analyzed by AEDs as "shock advised" as either VT or VF.

Of 188 reports, 37 fulfilled the study criteria. Decedents were mostly male (95 percent) and 36 years of age (± ten years). The time from discharge to collapse was less than one minute in 11 decedents, one to five minutes in 14 decedents, and six to 15 minutes in 12 decedents. Overall, the presenting rhythm was PEA or a bradyarrhythmia in 84 percent, sinus rhythm in 11 percent, and VT or VF in five percent. The two decedents with VT or VF collapsed within one minute of TASER discharge. The researchers concluded that the majority of rhythms recorded in sudden, custodial death after application of a TASER ECD were PEA or bradyarrhythmia. They opined that their findings did not support electrically induced VT or VF as the primary mechanism, but they are consistent with metabolic, respiratory, and/or toxic effects.

Conducting a retrospective review of TASER ECD associated, non-traumatic deaths from 2001 to 2008, Swerdlow, Fishbein, Chaman, Lakkireddy, and Tchou (2009) examined the cases of 56 subjects who collapsed within 15 minutes of ECD discharge and analyzed the first reported cardiac arrest rhythm. The rhythm was VF in four of the subjects and bradyarrhythmia, asystole, or PEA in 52 subjects. None of eight subjects who collapsed during electrocardiograph monitoring had VF. Only one subject collapsed immediately after ECD discharge. That one death was the only one that featured characteristics typical of electrically induced VF. The time from collapse to first recorded rhythm was less than five minutes for 43 subjects. The researchers concluded that, following ECD discharge, immediate collapse was unusual, and VF was an uncommon presenting rhythm. Within the limitations of the study, they argued that their data did not support electrically induced VF as a common mechanism of sudden deaths.

Bozeman, Teacher, and Winslow (2012) reviewed a database of consecutive TASER ECD uses against criminal suspects from six separate sites. The case reports contained demographic information, ECD deployment details, diagrams showing probe impact locations, and injuries sustained. Three investigators independently reviewed the case reports to identify incidents with paired anterior thoracic probe sites that could potentially produce transcardiac discharge. Of 1,201 cases studied, 179 included probe deployments with the potential for transcardiac discharge, which represented 14.9 percent of all TASER ECD uses and 22.0 percent of uses in probe mode. They found no report of immediate fatal collapse, and none of the uses resulted in immediate collapse that would suggest cardiac arrhythmia.

Case study reports have suggested temporal correlation between the use of ECDs and adverse cardiac effects. In a letter to the editor of the *New England Journal of Medicine*, Kim and Franklin (2005) described a case history report wherein officers used a TASER ECD to subdue an adolescent male, who subsequently collapsed. They reported that paramedics found the adolescent in VF and began performing cardiopulmonary resuscitation within two minutes after the collapse. After four shocks from a defibrillator and administration of epinephrine, atropine, and lidocaine, they restored a perfusing rhythm. They reported, also, that the adolescent made a nearly complete recovery and was discharged from the hospital several days later.

The letter has received a lot of attention from critics of TASER technology. However, what the letter did not report was that immediately following the subdual of the violently resisting adolescent, paramedics examined him and found a normal pulse and respirations. About 14 minutes later, the young man experienced cardiorespiratory collapse. VF did not occur until at least 20 minutes following the application of the shock and after medical interventions, including several cardiac shocks and the administration of atropine and epinephrine (Kroll, Calkins, and Luceri, 2007).

In a case study report, Richards, Kleuser, and Kluger (2008) described a cardioversion of atrial fibrillation to sinus rhythm in a patient after the delivery of a shock from an X26. The patient had presented to the emergency department in the custody of police. He had fled from officers and hidden in a lake for approximately 40 minutes. Officers brought him to the hospital because of concern for hypothermia. The initial evaluation by the emergency physicians found him to have an irregular pulse rate and a temperature of 89°F. His toxicology screen was positive for cocaine and amphetamines. His ECG showed atrial fibrillation, with a rapid ventricular response of 145 BPM. A cardiology consultant observed the patient to be in atrial fibrillation.

At the conclusion of the cardiologist's interview, the patient became increasingly agitated. He began ripping off all his monitoring electrodes, and he attempted to remove his intravenous line. He became threatening to the hospital staff and to the police officer who accompanied him. The police officer delivered one shock with an X26 in drive stun mode to the left anterior chest. Doctors checked the patient's pulse and found it to be in a rapid but regular rhythm. An ECG was performed immediately, which showed the patient to be in sinus tachycardia approximately two minutes following the application of the ECD.

The authors noted that spontaneous cardioversion from atrial fibrillation resulting from β-blocker therapy and even the act of voiding has been observed in patients. They concluded that it was plausible that the patient's cardioversion was related to the TASER ECD discharge, or to his treatment with β-blockers, or to spontaneous cardioversion from increased physical stress when he became combative.

Baldwin, Nagarakanti, Hardy, Jain, Borne, England, Nix, Daniels, Abide, and Glancy (2010) reported a case study of a 20-year-old man who suffered an acute MI after officers subdued him with a TASER ECD. The infarction was diagnosed by ECG, and troponin I levels were elevated, peaking at 10.73 ng/mL. Toxicology was negative for alcohol or drugs, but he did have high blood pressure and high cholesterol levels. Although the pathogenesis of the injury was uncertain, the authors suggested that transient spasm of the right coronary artery following the application of the ECD was a likely explanation.

Naunheim, Treaster, and Aubin (2010) reported a case study of a 17-year-old man who was intoxicated and violent. Officers shocked him in the anterior chest with a TASER ECD. Officers quickly observed that he was cyanotic and apneic. Within four minutes, paramedics arrived and found him in VF. They defibrillated him three times on the way to the hospital. On arrival at the hospital, he was in VF and his toxicology was positive for cannabis. His alcohol level was 235 mg/dL. Following aggressive treatment and hypothermia therapy, he recovered.

In a series case history study, Zipes (2012) reported eight people who suffered cardiac arrhythmia shortly following application of an X26. Seven of those cases resulted in the death of the individual, and one individual survived. All of the individuals received shocks with probes in a transcardiac configuration. On autopsy, pathologists discovered several victims had structural heart disease and/or had elevated blood alcohol concentrations. Three toxicology reports were positive for marijuana, and one was positive for medications for a seizure disorder. Zipes concluded that the use of a TASER ECD in the presence of structural heart disease and/or alcohol intoxication induced VT or VF. Zipes has been criticized for his interpretation of the medical evidence (Heegaard, Halperin, and Luceri, 2013), his representation of the facts (Ho and Dawes, 2013), and his characterization of the deceased as clinically healthy (Vilke, Chan, and Karch, 2013).

Pacemakers and Implantable Cardioverter-Defibrillators
In seven studies and case reports involving the effect of TASER technology on pacemakers and ICDs, researchers have found no evidence of damage to those devices. Additionally, they have found no evidence that a pacemaker or ICD has delivered inappropriate therapy following use of a TASER ECD. However, evidence does exist to suggest that longer than normal discharges of the ECD could result in a therapeutic shock from an ICD.

Researchers at the Defence Science and Technology Laboratory (2003) evaluated the risk that an M26 posed to people wearing pacemakers or other similar implantable devices. They noted that at the time of the study there were no reports of people wearing pacemakers being subjected to the discharge of a TASER ECD, and there was little independent information that dealt directly with the effects of a TASER discharge on the function of ICDs. The few existing studies showed that there were some effects on the functionality of the pacemaker, such as reversion to fixed asynchronous mode, but the effect was temporary and ceased when the ECDs were removed. They surmised that the effects of a TASER discharge on ICDs were likely to be similar to those on cardiac pacemakers. The nature of the cardiac rhythm sampling process, that is two samples approximately ten seconds apart, meant that application of a TASER ECD for the standard five seconds was unlikely to result in inappropriate therapy delivery. They also noted that the age profile of cardiac pacemaker recipients was significantly different from both the general population and that of persons arrested in situations where an ECD might be deployed. They determined that the probability of an individual wearing a pacemaker being present in such a situation was likely to be much lower than the incidence of pacemakers in the population, which was approximately 0.45 percent.

Calton, Cameron, Massé, and Nanthakumar (2007) noted that detection of TASER ECD discharges by ICDs had been described, but the effects of duration of TASER discharge and ICD detection and therapy had not been established. The researchers hypothesized that a longer duration of energy might lead to shocks from the defibrillator. They tested their hypothesis in a pig implanted with an ICD. They delivered TASER discharges for five and 15 seconds across the chest, using an M26. When they delivered the discharge for five seconds, the ICD detected energy as VF, but it delivered no shock. During charging of the capacitors, the ICD confirmed that the episode had terminated. However, when the energy was delivered for 15 seconds, the ICD detected energy as VF and delivered a shock. As the energy continued, the device redetected VF, and, even though the energy delivery had stopped during capacitor charging, the ICD delivered a second shock because the device was in committed mode during the second therapy for VF. They concluded that, in patients with more recent devices, 15-second shocks could result in ICD discharge. Second, because most ICDs were committed to deliver a shock after the first VF therapy, inappropriate shock might be delivered during sinus rhythm, even after energy was no longer being delivered. Finally, with older ICD models that have only committed shock delivery, even a short burst of energy delivery could result in inappropriate ICD discharges.

ICDs are known to be susceptible to malfunction from electromagnetic interference, so Lakkireddy, Khasnis, Antenacci, Ryshcon, Chung, Wallick, Kowalewski, Patel, Micochova, Kondur, Vacek, Martin, Natale, and Tchou (2007) implanted nine pacemakers and seven ICDs in pigs. They then applied a series of three standard five-second TASER discharges across the generators in the pigs' chests. They observed that mean pacing thresholds, sensing thresholds, pacing impedances and defibrillation coil impedances of the ICD leads were similar before and after the shocks. The devices aborted shock delivery in all tests as tachycardia detection abruptly terminated at the end of the five-second discharges. The researchers observed that the X26 discharges did not affect the short-term functions of implantable pacemakers and defibrillators even when the TASER probes were placed to sandwich the pulse generator.

Khaja, Govindarajan, McDaniel, and Flaker (2008) installed pacemakers in four pigs. They placed the pigs under anesthesia and exposed them to multiple shocks every three minutes from an M26, an X26, and another brand name ECD. The researchers recorded intracardiac electrograms continuously during discharges. The researchers noted that the pulse generator recognized the discharges and sensed it as either high rate atrial or ventricular activity depending on which vector was more in line with the electric field created by the two TASER probes. They also noted that the discharges did not affect the native rhythm, did not conduct down the lead systems to cause extra systoles, and had no effect on paced rhythm.

Vanga, Bommana, Phil, Kroll, Swerdlow, and Lakkireddy (2009) reviewed the literature on pacemaker and ICD interactions with TASER ECDs and presented six new case reports. The authors noted that oversensing of TASER ECD discharges might cause noise reversion pacing in pacemakers and inappropriate detection of VF in ICDs. However, the nominal five-second discharge of TASER ECDs was sufficiently short that neither clinically significant inhibition of bradyarrhythmia pacing nor inappropriate ICD shocks had been reported. The current evidence indicated that ECD discharges did not have adverse effects on pacemakers and ICDs.

Using a numerical anatomical model, Leitgeb, Niedermayr, Nuebauer, and Loos (2012) constructed three different models of pacemaker patients and numerically inserted a digital model of a cardiac pacemaker. They calculated intracorporal electric field distributions for various hits with a commercial software package and ran simulations with various TASER probe locations. They concluded that even worst-case probe mode hits of the X26 should not cause damage or persisting malfunction of the pacemakers. However, X26-induced interference voltages are more than two orders of magnitude above pacemaker sensing levels and, hence, may lead to pacemaker capture effects. Induced interference with cardiac pacemaker function could be expected when applying X26 ECDs to the upper part of the body, including the abdomen, with both frontal and dorsal hits. Although sensing a single pulse should have no major impact, cardiac capture is more likely for repeated pulse series.

Haegeli, Sterns, Adam, and Leather (2006) reported on the first documented case of a patient with an ICD who had experienced a field application of a TASER ECD. A 51-year-old woman had undergone placement of a single-chamber ICD five years earlier. Law enforcement officers applied a shock from an M26 due to the woman's violent behavior. The probes struck her sternum, and the current was applied for five seconds. The woman suffered no immediate adverse effects. Two months later, she presented for a regularly scheduled follow-up. When technicians examined data recorded in the ICD, the counters revealed one episode of VF, which corresponded to the time of the application of the TASER device.

The initial intervals of the sensed intrinsic ventricular activations were 435 to 443 ms, which corresponded to sinus tachycardia of 135 to 138 BPM. This rhythm was followed by high-frequency, high-amplitude electrical signals with intervals between 138 and 275 ms, which corresponded to the time of energy delivery by the M26. The ICD interpreted the episode as VF, resulting in the capacitor charging for VF therapy. At the end of the charge phase, the device attempted to reconfirm VF, but by that time, the TASER pulses had finished, and the ICD was no longer detecting VF. The energy that the ECD delivered did not significantly alter the sinus tachycardia of the patient. Delivery of the pulses induced neither VT nor VF. Further interrogation of the defibrillator did not reveal any detrimental alteration in the leads or circuitry.

Cao, Shinbane, Gillberg, Saxon, and Swerdlow (2007) described an X26 application on a person with a pacemaker that demonstrated evidence of ECD-induced myocardial capture. During an examination, doctors reviewed the recorded data in the pacemaker in a 53-year-old man with a dual-chamber pacemaker. He had received two shocks from an ECD consisting of two probes delivered simultaneously. Assessment of the pacemaker's functions demonstrated normal sensing, pacing thresholds, and lead impedances. Stored event data revealed two high ventricular rate episodes that corresponded to the time of the application of the TASER ECDs. The report of ventricular myocardial capture raised the question as to whether the X26 could cause primary myocardial capture or capture only in association with cardiac devices that provide a preferential pathway of conduction to the *myocardium*.

Intracardiac electrograms from pacemakers and ICDs in human reports have suggested the possibility of rapid myocardial capture. Electromagnetic interference related to ECD use was also questioned. However, animal studies had shown no effects on such devices. In this case series analysis, Lakkireddy, Biria, Baryun, Berenbom, Pimentei, Emert, Kreighbaum, Kroll, and Verma (2008) sought to determine whether evidence of myocardial capture was evident in three human cases. The first case was of a 25-year-old male. He was diagnosed with schizophrenia, and he received a pacemaker for sick sinus syndrome. His aggressive behavior resulted in officers shocking him on his chest three times with a TASER ECD, but there was no evidence of electromagnetic interference behavior or rapid myocardial capture on the electrograms. The second case was of a 45-year-old male with dilated cardiomyopathy who had a dual chamber ICD. He received two shocks on his back without any evidence of ICD shocks, rapid myocardial capture or electromagnetic interference behavior. The third case was of a 56-year-old male with a single chamber ICD for ischemic cardiomyopathy. He received four TASER shocks to the front with no electrogram evidence of ICD shocks, electromagnetic interference behavior or rapid myocardial capture.

Another case study documented a 58-year-old man who made a routine clinic visit without any complaints. An ICD had been implanted 6 years earlier after he presented with syncope and was found to be inducible for VT. He had a prior MI and his left ventricular ejection fraction was 30 percent. At device interrogation he was found to have a non-sustained arrhythmia detection corresponding to the time he was arrested in an intoxicated state. A TASER ECD had been used during his arrest. The electrogram demonstrated nonphysiologic noise consistent with ECD application. Oversensing was observed on both the atrial and ventricular channels. At ICD confirmation prior to the shock, the TASER ECD was off, thus, no ICD shock was delivered (Paninski, Marshall, and Link, 2013).

RESPIRATORY EFFECTS OF TASER ECDs

Human model experiments failed to produce evidence of an immediate cardiac effect to explain arrest-related sudden deaths following the application of TASER ECDs, so researchers began to explore other possible mechanisms. While testing for cardiac effects, researchers had noted that breathing was sometimes interrupted during application of TASER discharges in swine model experiments. One theory of potentially harmful effects in humans suggested that electric impulses from the ECD affected the phrenic nerve, thereby disturbing muscle contractions in the diaphragm and impairing normal breathing. Resulting hyperventilation could lead to elevated serum pH, known as alkalosis, and hypoventilation could lead to lowered serum pH levels, or acidosis (Dawes, 2009).

Chan, Sloane, Neuman, Levine, Castillo, Vilke, Bouton, and Kolkhorst (2007) conducted a randomized controlled trial in 28 volunteers who underwent a standard five-second X26 discharge as part of their law enforcement training. The researchers monitored test subjects for tidal volume, respiratory rate (RR), minute ventilation, end-tidal carbon dioxide (CO_2), and blood oxygen (O_2) saturation at baseline, during, and at one, ten, 30, and 60 minutes after discharge. They also obtained arterialized capillary samples for pH, partial pressure of oxygen (pO_2), and partial pressure of carbon dioxide (pCO_2) at baseline and at one, ten, 30, and 60 minutes after discharge. They found that mean minute ventilation, tidal volume, and RR all increased at one minute after discharge and returned to baseline levels at ten, 30, and 60 minutes. Mean pH decreased at one minute and returned to baseline levels at ten, 30, and 60 minutes. They observed no differences in blood O_2 saturation, pO_2, end-tidal CO_2, or pCO_2 over time, and they saw no evidence of abnormal hypoxemia or hypoventilation.

Ho, Dawes, Bultman, Thacker, Skinner, Bahr, Johnson, and Miner (2007) subjected 52 volunteers to a 15-second application from a TASER ECD while those volunteers were wearing respiratory measurement devices. Thirty-four volunteers underwent a 15-second continuous exposure, and 18 underwent three five-second exposures. The researchers collected common respiratory parameters before, during, and after exposure. In the continuous application group, during exposure, the baseline mean tidal volume increased. After exposure, the baseline end-tidal CO_2 level decreased, and the baseline end-tidal O_2 level and the baseline RR increased. In the five-second burst group, during exposure, the baseline mean tidal volume increased. After exposure, the baseline end-tidal CO_2 level decreased, and the baseline end-tidal O_2 level and the baseline RR increased. The researchers concluded that prolonged application did not impair respiratory parameters.

Dawes, Ho, Johnson, and Miner (2007a) examined venous blood gases and blood chemistries in 18 subjects who were exposed to a field deployable X26 modified to allow a 15-second discharge. They ran venous blood samples to obtain pH, pCO_2, pO_2, bicarbonate, lactate, sodium, and potassium immediately preceding the experiment and immediately after the exposure. The respiratory data showed no significant changes before, during, or after exposure except for an increase in RR during the exposure. Blood chemistries showed a statistically significant decrease in potassium, pCO_2 and bicarbonate, and a statistically significant increase in pO_2, and lactate. The data showed no significant change in pH or sodium post-exposure.

Ho, Lapine, Joing, Reardon, and Dawes (2008) applied an X26 in drive stun mode to the trapezius muscle of one volunteer to determine whether the electric current travelled to the phrenic nerve resulting in diaphragmatic paralysis or travelled up the spinal cord to the respiratory center of the brain. The researchers applied a 10-second drive stun while observing the diaphragm through ultrasonography. They observed no evidence of paralysis of the diaphragm.

Ho, Dawes, Reardon, Moscati, Gardner, and Miner (2008) enrolled 21 volunteer law enforcement officers and physicians who were attending training in the use of TASER ECDs to undergo two five-second drive stun applications with a one-second rest period between shocks of an X26. All applications were delivered either to the trapezius muscle or to lower extremities. They observed the diaphragm through ultrasonography and noted that it moved consistent with normal breathing in all subjects.

Dawes, Ho, Johnson, Lundin, Janchar, and Miner (2008), noting that previous studies regarding the possible effects of TASER shocks on breathing involved thoraco-abdominal exposure, tested the effects of exposure transversely across the chest. They placed one electrode from an X26 midline about one inch below the sternal notch. They placed the second electrode about 12 inches below the first and left of midline from one to seven inches. They measured RR, tidal volume, end-tidal CO_2 and end-tidal O_2 of 15 volunteers and then subjected each volunteer to a continuous 10-second discharge. They observed that the volunteers experienced an increase in RR, minute volume, and end tidal O_2. The volunteers also experienced a decrease in tidal volume and end-tidal CO_2 during the exposure. After exposure, tidal volume and minute ventilation remained elevated.

Dawes, Ho, Orozco, Vogel, Nelson, and Miner (2010) tested the X3, the latest generation ECD that has the capability of firing three cartridges in a semi-automatic mode, to determine its metabolic, neuro-endocrine, and respiratory effects. A master instructor applied an X3 to the anterior thorax of test subjects with either one or two cartridges. Each subject received a ten-second exposure. Fifty-three subjects completed the study. Researchers reported no important changes in vital signs and no evidence of impairment to breathing.

VanMeenen, Lavietes, Cherniack, Bergen, Teichman, and Servatius (2011) conducted an experiment on 25 people to determine whether a shock from an X26 impaired the ability to breathe during exposure. Participants were either equipped with alligator clips on their clothing, or they received an ECD discharge to their back. Respiration was measured through changes in flow and temperature continuously for 20 seconds before the exposure, during the exposure, and for 20 seconds post-exposure. Pulse oximetry was continuously measured during the same period. Self-report measures were taken immediately post-exposure. Of the 25 people who participated, two were excluded due to system failures resulting in exposures of less than two seconds. Although they were actively trying to breathe, most participants showed an absence of orderly tidal breathing. Inspiratory flow approached zero during the ECD exposure, and expiratory flow severely decreased. Sound recordings indicated that many of the participants with significant expiratory flow were also vocalizing. Normal breathing resumed after the cessation of the ECD exposure.

METABOLIC EFFECTS OF TASER ECDS

Human model experiments with TASER ECDs produced no evidence of direct cardiac effects, and the theory of death by direct electrical stimulation failed to explain collapses that occurred several minutes to several hours after discharge. Researchers began to explore the possibility that the TASER discharge could lead to delayed cardiovascular collapse by stimulating the neuroendocrine system and producing adverse metabolic effects. When exposed to TASER ECD discharges, the sympathetic-adrenal-medulla (SAM) axis and the hypothalamus-pituitary-adrenal (HPA) axis of the neuroendocrine system activate to cope with the induced stress reaction (Kunz, Groves, and Fischer, 2012).

The SAM axis causes the brain to send signals to the adrenal glands, which then release stored epinephrine to initiate the fight or flight response. Epinephrine increases the rate and strength of heart contractions, which is useful in short-term struggles, but it can also cause myocardial ischemia, arrhythmias, hyperthermia and lactic acidosis. The HPA axis causes the brain to signal the pituitary glands to release ß-endorphins and adrenocorticotropic hormone (ACTH). ß-endorphins reduce the pain from a fight, and ACTH helps to increase blood volume (Dawes and Kroll, 2009). The results of stimulation of the SAM and HPA axes, such as lactic acidosis, hyperthermia, and myocardial constriction bands, are common in arrest-related sudden deaths and in medical settings where law enforcement personnel are not present (Hick, Smith, and Lynch, 1999).

Animal Model Studies
Jauchem, Sherry, Fines, and Cook (2006) exposed six anesthetized pigs to repeated exposures of the X26 for five seconds, followed by a five-second period of no exposure continuously for three minutes. In five of the animals, after a one-hour delay, they added a second three-minute exposure period. The researchers observed some similarities in blood sample changes with previous studies of muscular exercise. They reasoned that problems concerning biological effects of repeated TASER pulse exposures might be related not directly to the electric output *per se*, but rather to the resulting contraction of muscles, related interruption of respiration, and subsequent sequelae. Transient increases in hematocrit, potassium, and sodium were consistent with previous studies of muscle stimulation or exercise.

Dennis, Valentino, Walter, Nagy, Winners, Bokhari, Wiley, Joseph, and Roberts (2007) anesthetized 11 pigs (six experimental and five controls) and exposed the experimental pigs to two 40-second discharges across the torso from an X26. The researchers obtained blood gases and electrolyte levels at five, 15, 30, and 60 minutes and 24, 48, and 72 hours post-discharge. The researchers observed two deaths immediately after TASER exposure from acute onset VF. In the surviving animals, the TASER discharge affected the acid-base status at the five-minute point and throughout the 60-minute monitoring period. Five minutes post-discharge, central venous serum pH decreased from baseline. Bicarbonate levels significantly decreased from baseline, and pCO_2 increased significantly from baseline. Researchers also observed a significant increase in lactate. All values returned to normal by 24 hours post-discharge in the surviving animals.

Esquivel and Bir (2008) performed a controlled hemorrhage on three male swine to induce tachycardia, hypotension and catecholamine release as compensatory mechanisms. They used one additional animal to study the effects of the stress alone. They warmed the animals to bring their core temperature to 108°F and exposed them to discharges from an ECD 20 times, at four sets of five exposures, in 30 minutes. They continuously monitored cardiac and pulmonary parameters, and they collected blood samples before and after each set of exposures and at one-hour intervals for four hours. As expected, the heart rate remained elevated for the entire study for all animals. The baseline pH, pCO_2, and lactate values were within the normal average values previously reported for swine. Serum pH decreased slightly after hemorrhage for all in the exposed group, and all three pigs in the exposed group became acidotic during the exposures. Blood lactate increased above normal after the hemorrhage and increased further after each set of exposures. Compared to a previous study in which the same device was applied on healthy, anesthetized swine, these animals were more acidotic and had a greater increase in blood lactate.

In a previous study of anesthetized swine, 18 repeated exposures from an X26 resulted in acidosis and increases in blood electrolytes (Jauchem, et al., 2006). Jauchem, Cook, and Beason (2008) examined the effects of more typical exposures. They exposed ten swine to three shocks (five seconds of exposure followed by five seconds of no exposure, repeated three times) and monitored blood factors for three hours following exposure. They observed transient increases in blood glucose, lactate, sodium, potassium, calcium, and pCO_2. However, they noted that these increases were consistent with studies of muscle stimulation in dogs and exercise in humans. Serum pH decreased immediately following exposure but rapidly returned to normal levels.

Jauchem, Beason, and Cook (2009) investigated the effects of exposures to a waveform similar to the X26 pseudo-monophasic waveform but without the initial arc phase. They anesthetized ten pigs ranging in weight from 56.8 to 63.8 kg and exposed them to the modified waveform for either 30 or 60 seconds. They placed one probe approximately five cm to the right of the midline approximately 13 cm above the xiphoid process. They placed the other probe approximately seven cm left of the umbilicus. They continuously monitored the pigs' heart rates, RR, and pulse oximeter O_2 saturation. They observed transient increases in potassium and sodium, which were consistent with literature on studies of muscle stimulation or exercise. Serum pH significantly decreased after exposure, but subsequently returned to baseline levels. Despite the low serum pH immediately after exposure, all the animals survived. Lactate was highly elevated and remained increased at three hours. Serum myoglobin increased after exposure and remained elevated for the three-hour follow-up period. The researchers concluded that acidosis would appear to be one of the major concerns with long-duration exposures over a short period.

Jauchem, Seaman, and Klages (2009) sedated ten pigs to examine the effects of exposures to a C2, the civilian version ECD. They observed that applications of the C2 for 30 seconds resulted in extensive muscle contractions, significant increases in heart rate, hematocrit, pCO_2, lactate, glucose, and potassium, sodium, and calcium ions. They also observed significant decreases in blood O_2 saturation, pO_2, and pH. They noted that many of the changes were consistent with previous reports dealing with studies of muscle stimulation or exercise. However, the changes in blood pCO_2, pO_2, electrolytes, lactate, and pH were greater than in a previous study of three repeated five-second exposures to the X26 commonly used by law-enforcement personnel (Jauchem, Cook, and Beason, 2008). They concluded that potential detrimental metabolic effects due to use of the C2 might be more likely than limited intermittent applications of the X26.

Human Model Studies

Ho, Miner, Lakkireddy, Bultman, and Heegaard (2006) examined the effects of TASER ECD applications in resting adult volunteers to determine whether there was evidence of induced or direct cellular damage. Sixty-six volunteer human subjects underwent 24-hour monitoring after one standard application. The subjects had medical histories that included asthma, diabetes, gout, hypertension, hypercholesterolemia, mitral valve prolapse, hypothyroidism, congestive heart failure, previous MI, and cerebrovascular disease. The researchers collected blood samples before exposure, immediately after exposure, and again at 16 and 24 hours after exposure. The researchers analyzed blood samples for markers of skeletal and cardiac muscle injury and renal impairment. They found no significant change from baseline at any of the four times for serum electrolyte levels and the blood urea nitrogen/creatinine ratio. They observed an increase in serum bicarbonate and creatine kinase levels at 16 and 24 hours, and they noted an increase in serum lactate level immediately after exposure that decreased at 16 and 24 hours. Serum myoglobin level increased from baseline at all three times. They found no evidence of dangerous hyperkalemia or induced acidosis.

Bouton, Vilke, Chan, Sloane, Levine, Neuman, Levy, and Kolkhorst (2007) enrolled 21 volunteers to experience a single five-second TASER exposure. The researchers took baseline measurements before exposure and took measurements of minute ventilation, tidal volume, RR, end-tidal pO_2, serum pH, bicarbonate, and lactate for 60 minutes following exposure. They observed that serum pH decreased at one minute post-exposure but returned to baseline within ten minutes. Bicarbonate concentrations decreased at one minute and ten minutes post-exposure but returned to baseline within 30 minutes. Lactate concentrations increased at one minute and ten minutes post-exposure but returned to baseline within 30 minutes. The researchers concluded that a single five-second TASER exposure did not cause clinically significant indications of physiological stress that could be causally linked to sudden death.

Vilke, Sloane, Bouton, Kolkhorst, Levine, Neuman, Castillo, and Chan (2007) enrolled 32 healthy law enforcement officers to receive a five-second TASER ECD discharge. Before and for 60 minutes after exposure researchers measured end-tidal pCO_2, O_2 saturation, arterial blood for pH, pO_2, pCO_2, and lactate, and venous blood for bicarbonate and electrolytes. At one minute post-exposure, researchers observed that blood lactate increased from baseline returning to baseline at 30 minutes. Serum pH and bicarbonate decreased at one minute returning to baseline at 30 minutes. They observed no clinically significant or lasting significant changes in electrolyte, lactate, or pH levels.

Ho, Dawes, Lapine, Bultman, and Miner (2008) enlisted 21 volunteers to receive either one 15-second or two consecutive five-second drive stun applications from an X26. Eleven subjects received the longer application, and ten subjects received the shorter repeated applications. All applications were to the neck and shoulder area. The researchers obtained blood samples immediately following exposure and again at eight hours and 24 hours after exposure. They found no significant changes from baseline in blood urea nitrogen/creatinine ratio or serum potassium levels. They did observe a significant decrease in serum lactate at the eight-hour level. The researchers concluded that their data did not support theories of worsening physiologies following drive stun applications of the X26.

Ho, Dawes, Bultman, Moscati, Skinner, Bahr, Reardon, Johnson, and Miner (2007) monitored 44 subjects after an anaerobic exercise regimen followed by a 15-second TASER ECD application to determine whether prolonged applications had significant physiologic effects on acidotic humans. They collected venous blood before and after exercise to verify acidosis and again after exposure to evaluate effect. They also included a control sample that exercised but underwent sham exposures for comparison. The researchers analyzed samples for markers of cardiac muscle injury and acidosis. The researchers discovered that there was a similar decrease in pH after exercise in both the controls and the exposed subjects. Following sham and real exposures, researchers observed similar increases in pCO_2, pO_2, and serum lactate in control and exposed groups. They noted that markers of acidosis and cardiac injury were similar among acidotic subjects who underwent both sham and real prolonged exposure. They concluded that prolonged TASER ECD exposure in humans did not appear to have an effect with regard to worsening acidosis that was already present.

Vilke, Sloane, Suffecool, Neuman, Castillo, Kolkhorst, and Chan (2007) enlisted eight volunteers to receive one five-second TASER activation after rigorous exercise. The researchers took baseline cardiovascular measurements and blood samples before the test subjects exercised to 85 percent of maximum heart rate. Researchers took a second set of blood samples when subjects reached the predicted heart rate. The subjects then received a five-second ECD exposure. The researchers rechecked blood samples at one, ten, 30, and 60 minutes post-exposure. Blood measures included arterialized capillary samples for pH, pCO_2, pO_2, bicarbonate, and lactate. Serum pH and bicarbonate both decreased from baseline to post-exercise while lactate increased. Bicarbonate measures were lower at one minute and ten minutes post-exposure when compared to post-exercise before starting to increase toward baseline measures at 30 minutes post-exposure. Serum pH returned to baseline levels by 30 minutes post-exposure, and bicarbonate and lactate returned to baseline levels by 60 minutes post-exposure. The researchers reported that the changes were not clinically significant.

To determine whether a 15-second discharge from an X26 caused acidosis, hyperkalemia, or serum lactate change in exhausted humans, Ho, Dawes, Bultman, Moscati, Janchar, and Miner (2009) enrolled 38 volunteers to undergo an exercise protocol to exhaustion. The researchers drew blood from the volunteers pre-exercise and again when they could no longer perform the exercises at the designated pace. They then applied a 15-second discharge from an X26. They drew blood immediately after the exposure, and a fourth time between 16 and 24 hours after exposure. The researchers tested the blood samples for pH, pCO_2, potassium, and lactate. Median pre-exposure serum pH decreased following exercise, decreased again following exposure, and recovered to normal at 24 hours. The median pCO_2 increased after exercise, decreased immediately after exposure, and returned to pre-test levels at 24 hours. Lactate increased immediately after exercise and immediately after exposure, but decreased to normal at 24 hours. Serum potassium increased immediately after exercise, decreased following exposure, and recovered to normal levels at 24 hours. The researchers concluded that a prolonged exposure from an X26 did not result in worsening acidosis or hyperkalemia, but it was associated with a small increase in serum lactate.

Vilke, Sloane, Suffecool, Kolkhorst, Neuman, Castillo, and Chan (2009) enrolled 25 healthy police volunteers to test the effects of a single exposure from a TASER ECD on markers of physiologic stress. The volunteers exercised to 85 percent of maximum heart rate and then experienced a standard five-second TASER shock. Before and for 60 minutes after the TASER application the researchers measured arterialized blood for pH, pO_2, pCO_2, and lactate. Each volunteer then repeated the exercise and data collection without TASER activation. The researchers observed, after adjusting for multiple comparisons, that the TASER-exposed group had significantly higher systolic blood pressure, but they observed no other significant differences between the two groups in any other measure at any time. From their observations they concluded that a single five-second exposure from a TASER ECD following vigorous exercise did not result in clinically significant changes in parameters of physiologic stress.

In many cases of arrest-related sudden death, especially in cases of ExDS or sympathomimetic drug toxicities, the deceased are found to be hyperthermic. Dawes, Ho, Johnson, Lundin, Janchar, and Miner (2007) examined whether a TASER ECD discharge caused an increase in core body temperature in non-environmentally stressed resting adults. They enrolled 21 volunteers to swallow a telemetric temperature recording capsule, and they recorded the volunteers' core body temperature every 15 seconds on a device attached to the test subjects' waists. Researchers then exposed the subjects to a 15-second continuous discharge from the X26. There was no change in temperature after the exposure in the majority of patients. One patient had a 0.2°F increase at 20 minutes, and three patients had a 0.1°F decrease in temperature at ten minutes or 20 minutes.

Dawes, Ho, Johnson, Lundin, Janchar, and Miner (2008) exposed 17 non-environmentally stressed resting adult human volunteers to a 15-second continuous discharge from an X26. A control group of ten subjects conducted usual activities of daily living. The researchers measured core body temperature every 15 seconds via a swallowed telemetric temperature measuring device. They found that the discharge from the X26 did not cause an elevation in core body temperature.

Moscati, Ho, Dawes, and Miner (2010) questioned whether ECD use might have different physiologic effects on alcohol intoxicated subjects. They enrolled 26 volunteer subjects, 22 as test subjects and four as controls. After they had obtained baseline blood samples, the researchers gave mixed drinks to the test subjects in a controlled setting to achieve a blood alcohol level of 0.08 mg/dL. The researchers drew blood samples after the subjects reached the target alcohol level. They then exposed the subjects to a 15-second TASER discharge. They drew blood samples immediately afterward and again at 24 hours.

They analyzed the samples for markers of acidosis and troponin I. They observed no difference between groups for baseline pH, pCO_2, lactate, or troponin I. Following intoxication, but prior to ECD exposure, there was no difference between groups in blood alcohol or repeat measures of pH, pCO_2, and lactate. Following exposure, there was a small drop in pH, a non-significant rise in pCO_2, and a rise in lactate. At 24-hour post-exposure, there was again no difference between controls and study groups in pH, lactate, and troponin I. There was a statistically significant change in pCO_2. The researchers concluded that intoxicated adults with prolonged exposure demonstrated small transient increases in measures of acidosis, but the increased acidosis self-corrected and was not clinically significant.

Dawes, Ho, Johnson, and Miner (2007b) noted that the electrical current from an X26 stimulated afferent sensory neurons, the neurons that cause pain, and efferent motor neurons, the neurons that cause skeletal muscle contractions. They also recalled speculation in the lay press and in medical literature that a TASER ECD discharge might induce neuroendocrine effects that could predispose subjects to delayed arrhythmias and sudden death. They compared the neuroendocrine effects of the X26 to oleoresin capsicum (OC) spray by enrolling ten volunteers to receive either a five-second exposure from the X26 with probes fired in the back or a two-second spray of OC spray to the eyes. The researchers collected salivary samples before exposure and at ten, 20, and 60 minutes after exposure and analyzed the samples for alpha-amylase, a surrogate for SAM axis stimulation, and cortisol, a surrogate for HPA axis stimulation.

Researchers observed a 173 percent increase in alpha-amylase in the OC spray group at ten minutes compared to an eight percent decrease in the ECD group. At one hour, alpha-amylase was 44 percent over baseline in the OC spray group and nine percent over baseline in the ECD group. There was an 89 percent increase in cortisol in the OC spray group at 20 minutes and a 90 percent increase in the ECD group. At one hour, cortisol was 15 percent over baseline in the OC spray group and 68 percent over baseline in the ECD group. The researchers concluded that the results suggested a significantly greater level of activation of the SAM axis cascade with OC spray compared to the X26. Overlapping confidence intervals precluded a definitive statement about the other measurements, but they opined that the results did not suggest a greater activation of the stress cascade by the X26 than by OC spray.

Dawes, Ho, and Miner (2009) tested the relative effects of the X26, OC spray, a cold-water tank immersion, and a defensive tactics drill on the human stress response. They enrolled 53 volunteers to conduct the experiment, but later excluded one due to a recent injury. They randomized the subjects to one of four interventions. Subjects received either a five-second exposure from an X26 with the probes fired into the back, a five-second spray of OC spray to the eyes, a 45-second exposure of the hand and forearm in a 0°C cold water tank, or a one-minute defensive tactics drill. The researchers observed that alpha-amylase had the greatest increase from baseline at ten to 15 minutes with the defensive tactics drill. Cortisol had the greatest increase at 15 to 20 min with OC spray. Cortisol remained most elevated at 40 to 60 minutes in the defensive tactics drill group. The researchers concluded that their data suggested physical exertion during custodial arrest might be most activating of the human stress response, particularly the SAM axis, and that the X26 was not more activating of the stress response than other uses of force.

Ho, Dawes, Cole, Hottinger, Overton, and Miner (2009) enrolled the assistance of 40 volunteers to determine whether exposure to a shock from an X26 on exhausted humans caused worsening acidosis compared with continued exertion. The researchers obtained medical histories and baseline pH and lactate values from the volunteers. They then divided the volunteers into four groups. One control group consisted of exertion only, and one control group consisted of X26 exposure only. One experimental group consisted of exertion plus X26 exposure, and the second experimental group consisted of exertion plus additional exertion. The researchers drew blood samples after each exertion effort and each X26 exposure. They repeated the blood draws every two minutes for 20 minutes. They found no statistical differences between X26 exposure groups at baseline or between exertion groups immediately upon completion of an exercise protocol. However, the X26 exposure control group had higher pH and lower lactate values at all times after exposure compared with the exertion only control group. Following the exertion protocol, there were no significant differences in the pH or lactate values between the experimental groups at any time. The researchers concluded that X26 exposure did not worsen acidosis in exhausted humans differently than continued exertion.

Previous researchers had opined that temporal relationships between arrest-related sudden deaths and the use of TASER ECDs might be related to acute stress cardiomyopathy induced by high levels of catecholamines. Ho, Dawes, Ryan, Lundin, Overton, Zeiders, and Miner (2009) enrolled 60 volunteers and randomized them into five groups: (1) a 150 meter sprint simulating flight from law enforcement officers, (2) 45 seconds of hitting and kicking a heavy bag to simulate physical combat, (3) a ten-second exposure from an X26, (4) a canine training exercise of approximately 30 seconds, or (5) OC spray exposure to the face. Researchers drew blood samples to determine baseline levels of epinephrine, norepinephrine, dopamine, and total catecholamines. Each volunteer then participated in one of the five tasks. Researchers drew blood samples for catecholamines, lactate, and serum pH within 30 seconds after completion of the task and every two minutes for ten minutes. The researchers determined that there was no difference in baseline catecholamine levels between the groups. After the tasks, the highest median was the heavy bag group followed by the sprint group. The canine group was next, the X26 group was fourth, and the OC spray group was fifth. The pH and lactate results followed the same pattern, with pH the lowest and lactate the highest for the heavy bag, followed by the sprint group. The researchers concluded that an exposure from an X26 activated fewer catecholamines, produced lower levels of lactate, and had less of an effect on serum pH than physical combat, fleeing, and resisting a canine.

Expanding on previous research, Ho, Dawes, Nelson, Lundlin, Ryan, Overton, Zeiders, and Miner (2010) enlisted 66 volunteers in a law enforcement training academy and randomly assigned them to one of five study groups: (1) a 150 meter sprint and scale a 4-foot wall, (2) 45 seconds of maximal heavy bag exertion, (3) a ten-second exposure from an X26, (4) a 40-yard sprint and a 20-second fight with a law enforcement dog, or (5) OC spray exposure to the face. Sixty-two of the 66 volunteers completed their assignments. Additionally, the researchers included a sixth group of subjects who ran up and down two flights of stairs to simulate a common layperson activity for comparison. Researchers drew venous blood samples before and after the events. They continued sampling in two-minute intervals until 12 minutes post event and compared pH and lactate values between groups. The researchers determined: (1) the exertion groups of the heavy bag and the 150-meter sprint had lower pH and higher lactate after exposure than the other groups, (2) the exposures of the X26 and the OC spray had higher pH and lower lactate than the other groups, (3) volitional behaviors of resistance and fleeing induced the most profound levels of acidosis, (4) law enforcement tools and tactics did not induce acidosis to the same levels as volitional subject behavior, and (5) the common activity of briskly ascending and descending two flights of stairs caused acidosis physiology similar to a ten-second X26 application.

Ho, Dawes, Cole, and Miner (2008) enlisted four volunteers to experience a 20-second and one volunteer to experience a 30-second discharge to the thorax from the civilian TASER model, the C2. Researchers drew venous blood before, immediately after, and 24 hours post-discharge to analyze biomarkers of acidosis and cellular damage. Median baseline serum pH decreased following application, but returned to normal at 24 hours post-exposure. Median baseline potassium decreased following application, but returned to normal at 24 hours post-exposure. Median baseline lactate increased following application, but returned to normal at 24 hours post-exposure. Median baseline creatine phosphokinase decreased following application, but returned to normal at 24 hours post-exposure.

SUMMARY

High-risk group theory postulates that people with cardiovascular disease, people under the influence of drugs or who have a history of drug abuse, people intoxicated from alcohol, people who are under extreme psychological distress or who exhibit signs of ExDS, and people who are mentally ill or taking psychotropic medications are at higher risk of sudden death following application of a TASER ECD than people who do not suffer such infirmities. To date, research has not led to specification of a mechanism to explain why that should be true. Medical literature makes it clear that people in the high-risk group are already at higher risk of sudden death without police intervention. Human model studies have not demonstrated evidence of direct cardiac stimulation, cardiac damage, respiratory distress, or metabolic disturbance from the use of TASER ECDs that could create an increased risk of arrest-related sudden death.

CHAPTER 4

Testing High-Risk Group Theory

The present work is a retrospective open source research study of publicly available autopsy and toxicology reports. It is designed to compare the physiological attributes of high-risk group theory to two
groups of arrest-related sudden deaths, TASER ECD-proximate deaths
and non-ECD deaths. High-risk group theory postulates that elderly
people, young children, people with pre-existing cardiovascular disease, people with pacemakers and ICDs, people under the influence of
drugs or with a history of drug abuse, people intoxicated from alcohol
or with a history of chronic alcohol abuse, people under extreme psychological distress or who exhibit signs of ExDS, people who are mentally ill or who are taking psychotropic medications, people subjected
to repeated or multiple applications, and pregnant women are at a
heightened risk of arrested-related sudden death following application
of a TASER ECD.

Because there is no known incident of a pregnant woman dying
following the application of an ECD, and because medical records related to the six alleged fetal deaths following the use of an ECD are
exempt from disclosure under the Health Insurance Portability and Accountability Act, this study does not address the pregnancy portion of
high-risk group theory. Additionally, because multiple applications of
a TASER ECD implicate their use in all such deaths, a control or comparison group that is not subjected to a TASER ECD against which to
compare physiological differences does not exist. Consequently, this
study does not include an examination of the multiple applications as-
pect of high-risk group theory.

An arrest-related sudden death is a death that occurs following a collapse within 24 hours after the initial arrest or detention. The death must be unexpected, must not be the result of trauma or injury that a layperson could readily discern needs medical attention, and must follow a sudden change in clinical condition or the beginning of symptoms from which the deceased does not recover. The collapse that results in death must have occurred in the United States between January 1, 2006 and December 31, 2011.

Arrest-related sudden death includes the deaths of persons at the scene of an arrest or detention, deaths while in transit from an arrest scene in a police vehicle or ambulance, deaths of arrested subjects at medical facilities due to injuries or medical problems, and any death in a jail or detention facility if the change in clinical condition that leads to the death occurs within 24 hours of the initial arrest or detention. It encompasses deaths that occur while the person is in the physical custody of or under the physical restraint of law enforcement officers, including formal arrests, investigative detentions, and detentions for emergency medical care or mental health issues. Because medical science can keep people alive for long periods following a collapse, the death need not occur within 24 hours of the initial arrest or detention, but the change in clinical condition from which the person does not recover must occur with 24 hours of the initial arrest or detention.

Arrest-related sudden death does not include deaths from pre-existing conditions that are known to law enforcement officers at the time of the arrest or detention, deaths following a change in clinical state that occur more than 24 hours following a subject's initial arrest or detention, and deaths from physical trauma or injuries that are readily apparent or easily discernible to a layperson, such as officer involved shootings, deaths due to suicide, or obvious injuries due to falls or other accidents. The definition does include, however, deaths from internal injuries that are not easily detectible or discernible to the layperson, such as internal bleeding.

Because no database containing physiological data on arrest-related sudden deaths exists, this study first required construction of a sampling frame. A non-proportional stratified random sample of 300 publicly available autopsy and toxicology reports was obtained for study. To avoid researcher bias, two people with knowledge of medical terminology, but who were without an interest in the results of the study, coded the autopsy and toxicology reports for attributes relevant to examining high-risk group theory. Descriptive statistics, inferential statistics, and Qualitative Comparative Analysis were used to analyze the data and to compare designated attributes in deaths proximate to the use of TASER ECDs to deaths when no ECD was involved.

CONSTRUCTING A SAMPLING FRAME

No nationwide database exists on police use of force outcomes with incident-level data (Ho, 2009; White and Ready, 2010), and there is no nationwide data collection system to collect reliable and systematic incident-level data on arrest-related sudden deaths. Moreover, the five most commonly used sources for examining data related to in-custody deaths have substantial limitations (Borrego, 2011; White, et al., 2013). Most notably, they do not identify the deceased, which makes them of little use in identifying specific cases for the current research.

Without names or other identifying information, it was not possible to obtain individual autopsy records. Consequently, the first step was to construct a sampling frame that specifically identified individual cases of arrest-related sudden deaths. Information sources for previous studies on arrest-related deaths included news media sources (Ho, Heegaard, Dawes, Matarajan, Reardon, and Miner, 2009; White and Ready, 2009; White, et al., 2013; Williams, 2008), Internet searches (Strote, et al., 2005), police reports (Williams, 2008), and medical examiner records (Southall, et al., 2005; White, et al., 2013; Williams, 2008). Each source had advantages and limitations.

News media reports are readily available through commercial databases and Internet searches, and they are a principal source of reliable information. Reports often include the name of the deceased and information sufficient to establish whether the incident qualifies as an arrest-related sudden death. However, media outlets might not learn of an incident, they might choose not to publish a report on an incident, or they might publish details insufficient to identify the incident as an arrest-related sudden death. Newspapers in less populated municipalities and counties with small circulations often are not included in media databases, so their reports are not readily available for search and review.

Because individuals can publish web pages on any topic of interest, Internet searches can be used to identify some incidents on which the news media does not report. Additionally, web pages often contain more information than news media reports; however, the reliability of that information is often questionable. Information, rather than being an impartial reporting of the facts, might be promoting an agenda, and some web pages uncritically repeat misleading or incorrect information from other web sources. Nevertheless, cases discovered through web page searches can often be verified through other sources.

Police reports are useful for verifying cases that are already identified through other sources, but, because they are not searchable through commercial databases, police reports offer little help in identifying new cases. Nevertheless, if a questionable case requires clarification, reports can be obtained from some law enforcement agencies.

The one report on in-custody deaths relying strictly on medical examiner reports comes from Maryland, which has one chief medical examiner's office for the state. Therefore, the records are readily available for examination in one location. In many other states, however, individual counties have their own coroners or medical examiners. In Texas, more populated counties employ medical examiners. Less populated jurisdictions, however, generally contract for autopsy services with the larger counties' medical examiners or with private sector pathologists. In those less populated jurisdictions, a Justice of the Peace in the precinct within the county where the death occurs is the custodian of the record. Consequently, in such states autopsy and toxicology reports are not centrally located, and they are not searchable through commercial software applications. Of course, autopsy records are the most complete source of data related to the physiological attributes of the deceased.

This study adopted a multi-faceted approach to identify and confirm cases of interest. The first approach involved public news media searches through two commercial databases with extensive, though not necessarily concurrent, data sources, NewsLibrary®[3] and LexisNexis®[4]. Because news reports of arrest-related sudden deaths do not contain standardized language that would facilitate searches, this approach required using several different search terms and phrases. Appendix A, Search Terms, contains a list of 46 words and phrases searched for this study. Because it was common to locate news reports published long after an incident occurred, date parameters were extended to search for

---

[3] NewsLibrary® is a trademark of The McClatchy Company, registered in the United States. All rights reserved.

[4] LexisNexis® is a trademark of LexisNexis Group, registered in the United States. All rights reserved.

reports containing applicable search terms published from January 1, 2006 through August, 2013, but only incidents that occurred from January 1, 2006 through December 31, 2011 were included in this study.

Reports detailing circumstances that did not fit the definition of arrest-related sudden death, such as officer involved shootings or suicides, were excluded. Reports with circumstances that were questionable were preserved for comparison against information from other sources to determine whether the case should be excluded or recorded. Reports with circumstances fitting the definition of arrest-related sudden death were recorded in an Excel[5] spreadsheet for inclusion in the sampling frame.

The second approach involved searching the Internet through Bing[6] and Google[7] search engines. Using the same 46 search terms from Appendix A, this approach sought web pages referring to arrest-related sudden deaths that might not have appeared in news media reports. Although the reporting of facts might have been less reliable than in news media reports, cases were identified for verification through other sources. Again, only incidents that occurred from January 1, 2006 through December 31, 2011 were included in this study. Cases that did not fit the definition of arrest-related sudden death were excluded. Questionable cases were preserved for verification through other sources. Cases from apocryphal web sites that appeared to be arrest-related sudden deaths were preserved pending verification through other sources. Cases from reliable sites, such as news or government web pages, that fit the definition of arrest-related sudden death were recorded in the sampling frame.

The third approach involved a search of LexisNexis and FindLaw[8] databases for court decisions that involved wrongful death claims arising from in-custody deaths and excessive force claims. In their published opinions, judges often included a synopsis of the facts

---

of the case before applying the law and rendering a decision. Using the 46 search terms in Appendix A, this approach involved searching legal opinions for incidents that occurred from January 1, 2006 through December 31, 2011 that fit the definition of arrest-related sudden death, regardless of the date of the opinion. Cases that were not arrest-related sudden deaths were excluded. Questionable cases were compared against information from other sources to determine whether the case should be excluded or recorded. Cases that fit the definition of arrest-related sudden death were recorded in the sampling frame.

Each state has a designee to coordinate the collection of reports for the Deaths in Custody Reporting Program (DCRP). The fourth approach involved making a freedom of information request of each of the state coordinators for copies of all reports to the DCRP, excepting officer-involved shootings and suicides. Once the information reached the BJS, federal law prohibited the release of research or statistical information that was "identifiable to any specific private person for any purpose other than the purpose for which it was obtained (42 U.S.C. § 3789g(a))." Therefore, because it could not release the names of individuals, no information request was made of the BJS. However, until the information reached the BJS, the information collected by the coordinators was subject to the public information or freedom of information laws of the individual states (Burch, 2012). Although the reporting form, a CJ-11A, did not include detailed information about the incident, the reports could reveal cases for additional research and verification through other sources. In California and Texas, state laws mandate reports for every in-custody death. In those states the freedom of information request included data from each state's respective in-custody death databases. Once again, cases that did not fit the definition of arrest-related sudden death were excluded. Questionable cases were preserved for comparison against information from other data sources to determine whether the case should be excluded or recorded. Cases that fit the definition of arrest-related sudden death were recorded in the sampling frame.

All cases discovered from each of the four sources were cross-researched through the other sources to ensure proper selection for the sampling frame, and duplicate entries were deleted. This four-fold approach produced a nearly complete listing of arrest-related sudden deaths. Still, it is likely that some cases remained undiscovered.

PUBLIC INFORMATION LAWS AND AUTOPSY REPORTS

In many states, autopsy reports were publicly available for examination and study. However, state statutes prohibited the release of autopsy reports in Arkansas (Arkansas Codes Annotated 12-12-312(a)), Connecticut (Connecticut General Statutes § 19a-411), Illinois (410 Illinois Compiled Statutes 535/24), Louisiana (Louisiana Revised Statutes 44:19), Mississippi (Mississippi Code Annotated § 41-61-63), Nebraska (Nebraska Revised Statutes 84-712.05(2)), New Hampshire (New Hampshire Revised Statutes § 611-B:21), New Jersey (New Jersey Statutes 52:17B-92), New York (County Law § 677), Oregon (Oregon Revised Statutes § 192.501), Rhode Island (Rhode Island General Laws § 38-2-2), Virginia (Virginia Annotated Code § 32.1-283.B), Washington (Revised Code of Washington § 68.50.105), and West Virginia (Code of State Regulations 84 § 18.2). In Nevada (Opinion Number 82-12) and in South Carolina (Opinion Number 81-87), Attorney General Opinions prohibited disclosure of autopsy reports. In Massachusetts (*Globe Newspaper Company v. Chief Medical Examiner*, 404 Mass. 132 (1989)) and in Pennsylvania (*Johnstown Tribune Publishing v. Ross, 871 A.2nd 324* (2009)), state Supreme Court rulings prohibited the release of autopsy records. In Minnesota, autopsy records become public information 30 years after the death (Minnesota Statutes § 13.83). Consequently, cases from those states were recorded in the database, but no autopsy records were requested for deaths occurring in those states. When requested to provide reports, medical examiners and coroners in Montana and Wisconsin claimed confidentiality of autopsy reports, but no legal basis for the exemption was apparent.

In the rest of the states, autopsy records were generally available, but some exceptions still applied. For example, if an investigation, a prosecution, or a lawsuit was pending, the records were exempt from disclosure. Until the records were requested and the coroner or medical examiner responded to the request, there was no way to know whether an exception applied.

SELECTING A NON-PROPORTIONAL STRATIFIED RANDOM SAMPLE

Once the sampling frame of 1,060 cases was constructed and all of the cases from states that exempted autopsy reports from disclosure were listwise deleted only for purposes of extracting a sample, an Internet based random number generator that uses atmospheric noise instead of pseudo-random mathematical formulas was used to generate a random sequence of names.[9] A non-proportional stratified random sample was obtained by requesting autopsy reports for the first 150 non-ECD cases and the first 150 ECD-proximate cases from the randomly ordered list. When any coroner or medical examiner did not respond to a request, a second request was made. When there was no response to the second request, or when the coroner or medical examiner declined to release an autopsy or toxicology report, the autopsy report for the next name on the stratified list was requested, and so on, until 150 non-ECD reports and 150 TASER-proximate reports were received for coding.

DEFINITION OF TERMS

To ensure consistent interpretation and coding of autopsy and toxicology reports on the coding instrument, terms were given the following definitions:

> *Age* – The age for the person is the age in whole numbers that the coroner or medical examiner listed on the autopsy report.
>
> *Sex* – The sex for the person is the sex that the coroner or medical examiner listed on the autopsy report, either male or female.
>
> *Race/Ethnicity* – The race or ethnicity of the person is what the coroner or medical examiner listed as race and/or ethnicity on each report, Black or African/American, Hispanic, White or Caucasian, or Other for any other race or ethnicity.
>
> *Height* – The height in inches by whole numbers only as indicated by the coroner or medical examiner on the autopsy report.
>
> *Weight* – The weight in pounds by whole numbers only as indicated by the coroner or medical examiner on the autopsy report.
>
> *TASER ECD* – Any mention by the coroner or medical examiner in the autopsy report of the use of a TASER brand name ECD.
>
> *Cardiovascular Disease* – Any mention by the coroner or medical examiner in the autopsy report of any of the following conditions in the diagnosis section, as a cause of death, or as a contributing factor to the death. This list was not comprehensive, but it included cardiovascular diseases frequently described in autopsy reports.

---

[9] (Random.org at http://www.random.org/)

- Aortic stenosis
- Atherosclerosis
- Atrial fibrillation
- Atrial flutter
- Atrial myxoma
- Atrioventricular block
- Congestive heart failure
- Coronary artery disease
- Dilated cardiomyopathy
- Hypertrophic cardiomyopathy
- Hypoplasia
- Ischemic heart disease
- Long QT syndrome
- Mitral stenosis
- Mitral valve prolapse
- Multifocal atrial tachycardia
- Myocardial infarction
- Myocarditis
- Premature atrial contractions
- Restrictive cardiomyopathy
- Septal defects
- Sinus bradyarrhythmia
- Sinus tachycardia
- Supraventricular tachycardia
- Tricuspid regurgitation
- Tricuspid stenosis.

Pacemakers or Implantable Cardioverter-Defibrillators – Any mention by the coroner or medical examiner in the autopsy report that the deceased used a pacemaker, an ICD, or any other device to stimulate or regulate heartbeat, or that the deceased used a device designed automatically to convert fibrillation to a sinus rhythm.

Commonly Abused Recreational Drugs Present – Any mention by the coroner or medical examiner of a positive toxicology report for any of the following:

Amphetamines – Including methamphetamine, methylenedioxyamphetamine, methylenedioxymethamphetamine, and amphetamine.

Cocaine – Including cocaine and its metabolites, benzoylecgonine, ethylbenzoylecgonine and cocaethylene.

LSD – Including lysergic acid diethylamide and its metabolites, N-desmethyl-LSD, hydroxy-LSD, 2-oxo-LSD, and 2-oxo-3-hydroxy-LSD.

Marijuana – Including marijuana, tetrahydrocannabinol, or delta-9-tetrahydrocannabinol.

Opiates – Including heroin, diacetylmorphine, morphine, codeine, 3-monoacetylmorphine, or 6-monoacetylmorphine.

PCP – Including phencyclidine.

History of Drug Abuse – Any mention by the coroner or medical examiner of a history of abuse of any of the following:

Amphetamines – Including methamphetamine, methylenedioxy-amphetamine, methylenedioxymethamphetamine, and amphetamine.

Cocaine.

LSD – Lysergic acid diethylamide.

Marijuana – Including marijuana and hashish.

Opiates – Including heroin, diacetylmorphine, morphine, or codeine.

PCP – Phencyclidine.

Excited Delirium – Any mention by the coroner or medical examiner of excited delirium, agitated delirium, cocaine induced delirium, or drug induced delirium in the diagnosis section, as a cause of death, or as a contributing factor to the death.

Alcohol Present – Any mention by the coroner or medical examiner of the presence of alcohol or ethanol in the body of the deceased, any mention in the diagnosis section, listed as a cause of death, or listed as a contributing factor to the death.

History of Chronic Alcohol Abuse – Any mention by the coroner or medical examiner of a history of chronic alcohol abuse.

Mental Illness – Any mention by the coroner or medical examiner of a diagnosis of or a history of schizophrenia, bipolar disorder, or depression.

Psychotropic Medications – Any mention by the coroner or medical examiner of a positive toxicology report for any of the following. This list was not comprehensive, but it included medications frequently described in toxicology reports.

- Aripiprazole
- Chlorpromazine
- Clozapine
- Fluoxetine
- Olanzapine
- Fluphenazine
- Haloperidol
- Loperidone
- Loxapine
- Molindone
- Paliperidone
- Perphenazine
- Pimozide
- Quetiapine
- Risperidone
- Thioridazine
- Thiothixene
- Trifluoperazine
- Ziprasidone.

Respiration – Any mention by the coroner or medical examiner of any of the following in the diagnosis, as a cause of death, or as a contributing factor to the death:

- Anoxia
- Asphyxia

- Hypercapnia
- Hypoxia.

Metabolic Disorders – Any mention by the coroner or medical examiner of any of the following in the diagnosis, as a cause of death, or as a contributing factor to the death:

- Acidosis
- Alkalosis
- Hypercalcemia
- Hyperkalemia
- Hypernatremia

- Hypocalcemia
- Hypokalemia
- Hyponatremia
- Hypoxemia
- Ketoacidosis.

CODING AUTOPSY AND TOXICOLOGY REPORTS

To avoid rater bias, three people who were not involved in the research agreed to code the autopsy and toxicology reports. Two of the volunteers had previously been employed in health care services, although neither one was a physician or a pathologist. Therefore, a coding instrument and instructions on completing the coding instrument was developed to assist them. Appendix B is a copy of the coding instrument. The instrument consisted of labeled boxes that two of the three coders completed.

Appendix C contains the instructions for completing the instrument that the coders received. To aid the coders in recognizing the attributes of interest in the autopsy and toxicology reports, the instructions contained lists of cardiovascular diseases, drugs, and psychotropic medications that were likely to appear in the reports.

Two coders received copies of each of the autopsy reports redacted of personal identifying information. For demographic information, the coders recorded age, sex, race/ethnicity, height, and weight of each deceased as the coroner or medical examiner noted that attribute on the autopsy report. For the other categories—use of a TASER ECD, cardiovascular disease, pacemakers or implantable cardioverter-defibrillators, drugs present, history of drug abuse, excited delirium, mentally ill, and psychotropic medications—the coders scored the instrument with a dummy variable, either a 0 or a 1, indicating the absence (0) or the presence (1) of the attribute as indicated on the autopsy report. The instrument concluded with a space for the coders to note any concerns or questions they had concerning a given report. The third coder was to resolve any discrepancies that the first two coders, after consultation, could not reconcile. However, consultation with the first two coders reconciled all conflicts in the observations, so involvement of the third coder was never necessary.

CONCORDANCE

The coders were instructed on how to complete the instrument, and they were given a copy of the instructions before they began. The two coders scored the reports independently and did not see the other coder's instruments. To test whether the coders would score the reports consistently, they were presented with identical copies of 20 autopsy reports from the selected sample. After the coders had completed scoring the reports, each observation on the coding instruments was compared to ensure that the coders had consistently interpreted and coded the reports. The coding instrument contained 28 cells to record observations for each case, so there were 560 observations for the 20 trial coding. The coders scored only 16 of the 560 observations differently.

One conflict involved the height on a report. It was found that the height was listed differently in two places on the report. One coder recorded one height while the other coder recorded the other height. That conflict was resolved in favor of the taller height of 64 inches (5'4"). The shorter height would have resulted in the person having been only 54 inches tall (4'6"), which seemed abnormally short.

Five conflicts involved whether a TASER ECD had been used. In all five cases, one coder had scored the variable to indicate the use of an ECD, and the other coder had scored the variable to indicate the lack of an ECD. On consultation with the coders, it was discovered that one coder had seen terms indicating an "electroshock device," a "conducted energy weapon," or a similar term, but had not seen the brand name TASER. Consequently, that coder scored the observations as no use of an ECD. Because it was possible that some other brand name of ECD had been involved in an arrest-related sudden death, that coder was instructed that scoring the observation as no use of a TASER ECD was acceptable as long as a note was added to the instrument indicating that an ECD was used but there was no mention of the brand name. In that way, further research into each questioned case could resolve whether a TASER ECD had been used, and the report could be properly coded.

Four discrepancies involved the presence of cardiovascular disease. In one discrepancy, one coder had simply not noticed a reference in the report. In the other three discrepancies, one coder had seen a term not familiar to the coder and not included as a cardiovascular disease on the instruction sheet. Consequently, that coder scored the observation as no cardiovascular disease. The other coder recognized the reference as a cardiac disease and scored the observation as the presence of cardiovascular disease. These discrepancies were resolved in favor of scoring the observations as presence of cardiovascular disease, and the coder who had not before recognized the term as a cardiovascular disease agreed to score any later reference as the presence of cardiovascular disease.

The other six discrepancies were resolved as simple errors in observation. For those six discrepancies, whenever one was discovered, the coders were asked to revisit their scoring of that observation. In each case, one of the coders acknowledged having not seen the reference in the report and agreed to change the score on the instrument.

Upon completion of the trial scoring, the two coders received and scored the remaining 280 reports. The recorded scores on each instrument were compared for any discrepancies in the coding, and discrepancies were reconciled as in the trial process. Eventually, both coders agreed on the coding of all 8,400 observations, so the assistance of the third observer as a tie-breaker was never required.

Some data of interest were missing from the autopsy reports. The age of the deceased was missing from four reports and the race\ethnicity was missing from ten reports. All four missing ages were available from the other sources used to identify and verify cases for this study. For nine of the ten cases missing race/ethnicity data, the information was available from other sources related to the cases. For each of those cases, the information was known, but was not available to the coders. In those cases, the data were recorded in the database. In one non-ECD case, however, no race/ethnicity was identified in any of the sources, and freedom of information laws in the state where the death occurred prohibit release of police records that might have included the information. Therefore, the race/ethnicity in one case remained missing.

One surprising observation was the lack of any reference to the use of a TASER ECD in 30 autopsy reports for cases in which other sources had established their use. Although the autopsy reports contained descriptions of minor associated wounds, they contained no mention of an ECD. Nevertheless, because other sources established the use of an ECD, and because those cases were included in the study because of the use of an ECD, those cases were recorded as ECD-proximate deaths in the database. Additionally, in four cases selected for the sample that were originally identified as non-ECD deaths, autopsy reports revealed the use of a TASER ECD. Consequently, these cases were also recorded as ECD-proximate cases in the database, and substitute non-ECD cases were obtained for study.

STATISTICAL ANALYSIS

Three tiers of analysis were used in this study. First, descriptive statistics were used to describe the occurrence of arrest-related sudden deaths over the six years included in the study and to describe general differences between non-ECD and TASER ECD-proximate deaths. This analysis began with a description of trends derived from the entire sampling frame, including frequency analyses of the number of deaths year-to-year, the number of deaths by month of the year, and the number of deaths by state and by jurisdiction. Although not tenets of high-risk group theory, this trend analysis aids in the understanding of the prevalence of arrest-related sudden deaths in both the non-ECD and the ECD-proximate groups. Demographic data were reported on age, sex, and race/ethnicity. Age and sex data were available on nearly every case in the sampling frame because news media reports usually included that data, so analyses include both the population and the sample. Publicly available information sources often did not include the race or ethnicity of the deceased, so race/ethnicity analysis included data only from the sample. Age, sex, and race/ethnicity data were also compared to data from previous studies on arrest-related deaths.

Second, a Student's *t*-test was used to analyze the age parameter for both the population and the sample. A *t*-test is an appropriate test of significance for a small sample, two-group analysis (Grabetter and Wallnau, 2000). Significance was set at the $\acute{a} = 0.05$ level. Pearson's χ^2 test for independence was used to analyze individually the observed differences in the other physiological attributes of high-risk group theory—cardiovascular disease, pacemakers and ICDs, presence of drugs, history of drug abuse, excited delirium, presence of alcohol, chronic alcohol abuse, mental illness, and the use of psychotropic medications. Additionally, although not tenets of high-risk group theory, χ^2 was used to analyze sex and race/ethnicity. A χ^2 test for independence is an appropriate hypothesis test for non-parametric categorical data (Grabetter and Wallnau, 2000). Significance was set at the $\acute{a} = 0.05$ level. Logistic regression analysis (logit) was used to examine the extent to which physiological attributes affected the likelihood that an ECD was involved in an arrest-related sudden death. Logit is an appropriate hypothesis test for a categorical binary dependent variable (Grabetter and Wallnau, 2000). Although this approach is a non-traditional use of logit, setting the use of an ECD as the dependent variable for analysis (even though it is not dependent in the commonly used sense) permits an examination of each variable while controlling for the other variables, which the χ^2 analysis does not permit. Logit is measured in z-scores. Significance was set at the $|z| \geq 1.96$ level.

The third analytical tier, Qualitative Comparative Analysis (QCA), bridges the methodological gap between traditional quantitative multivariate statistical techniques and qualitative case study analysis (Ragin, 1987). QCA is a deterministic data reduction technique that uses Boolean algebra to simplify complex data structures. Popular in the social sciences, QCA is designed specifically for the study of cases as configurations or as combinations of set memberships (Ragin, 1999). This analytical method allows a researcher to focus on symptoms and behaviors as configurations, not as individual features that correlate, which is a serious limitation of traditional quantitative measures such as logistic regression analysis.

Arrest-related sudden deaths do not follow one specific path. They are often a product of multiple conjunctures of partial causes. Different causal paths can lead to the same outcome—in this case, death. The principal advantage of QCA lies in the recognition that multiple causes or multiple sets of causes can produce the same outcome and that any variable might or might not be causally related to an outcome depending upon context and the nature of the other variables of the case. Simply put, QCA can help to determine whether certain combinations of attributes predominate in deaths involving an ECD.

As a technique, QCA can summarize data, check coherence within the data, test existing theories and assumptions, test new ideas or theories, and elaborate new assumptions or theories (Rihoux, 2006). Several versions of QCA have emerged, including crisp set QCA (csQCA), fuzzy set QCA (fsQCA), and multiple value QCA (mvQCA). Dichotomous data, such as those used in this study, are common to csQCA.

In this study, the csQCA algorithm was used to analyze all 300 cases using software available from the University of Arizona.[10] The use of a TASER ECD was set as the outcome, and the other variables of cardiovascular disease, drugs present, excited delirium, alcohol present, and the combined variable of mental illness plus psychotropic medications were set as the causal conditions. No additional conditions or variables outside high-risk group theory were considered.

RESEARCH HYPOTHESES

From the results of previous arrest-related death studies, the average age of ECD-proximate deaths appeared to be slightly younger than all arrest-related deaths. Consequently, the hypothesis to test regarding age is:

H_{A1}: People who suffer an arrest-related sudden death following application of a TASER ECD are younger than those who suffer an arrest-related sudden death absent the use of a TASER ECD.

From the results of previous arrest-related studies, women constituted between 3.7 and 6.7 percent of all arrest-related deaths, but they constituted only 2.6 to 4.2 percent of ECD-proximate deaths. For the logit models, female was assigned a value of 0, and male was assigned a value of 1. The hypothesis to test regarding sex is:

H_{A2}: The frequency of a TASER ECD being involved in an arrest-related sudden death is not the same for men and women.

From the results of previous arrest-related studies, the percentage of Blacks in TASER ECD-proximate deaths was slightly higher than the percentage of Blacks on all arrest-related deaths. For the logit models, White was assigned a value of 0. All other races and ethnicities were assigned a value of 1. The hypothesis to test regarding race/ethnicity is:

---

[10] http://www.u.arizona.edu/~cragin/fsQCA/software.shtml

H$_{A3}$: The frequency of a TASER ECD being involved in an arrest-related sudden death is not the same for Whites and minorities (i.e., Blacks, Hispanics, and all other races and ethnicities).

Descriptions of the other variables of interest—cardiovascular disease, pacemaker or ICD, presence of drugs, history of drug abuse, excited delirium, presence of alcohol, history of chronic alcohol abuse, history of mental illness, and use of psychotropic medications—were described as dichotomous variables, either absent (0) or present (1). These analyses included data only from the sample because there was no way to predetermine whether news media reports were a reliable source of that information. Significance was set at the $\acute{a}$ = 0.05 level. The several hypotheses to test regarding these other predictor variables of interest are:

H$_{A4}$: The frequency of people with cardiovascular diseases suffering arrest-related sudden death is not the same for TASER ECD-proximate deaths and non-ECD deaths.

H$_{A5}$: The frequency of people with pacemakers or ICDs suffering arrest-related sudden death is not the same for TASER ECD-proximate deaths and non-ECD deaths.

H$_{A6}$: The frequency of people currently using drugs suffering arrest-related sudden death is not the same for TASER ECD-proximate deaths and non-ECD deaths.

H$_{A7}$: The frequency of people with a history of drug abuse suffering arrest-related sudden death is not the same for TASER ECD-proximate deaths and non-ECD deaths.

H$_{A8}$: The frequency of people exhibiting symptoms of ExDS suffering arrest-related sudden death is not the same for TASER ECD-proximate deaths and non-ECD deaths.

H$_{A9}$: The frequency of people intoxicated from alcohol suffering arrest-related sudden death is not the same for TASER ECD-proximate deaths and non-ECD deaths.

H$_{A10}$: The frequency of people with a history of chronic alcohol abuse suffering arrest-related sudden death is not the same for TASER ECD-proximate deaths and non-ECD deaths.

H$_{A11}$: The frequency of people with mental illness suffering arrest-related sudden death is not the same for TASER ECD-proximate deaths and non-ECD deaths.

H_{A12}: The frequency of people taking psychotropic medications suffering arrest-related sudden death is not the same for TASER
ECD-proximate deaths and non-ECD deaths.

CHAPTER 5

Research Findings

A thorough review of media data sources, the Internet, legal opinions, and data from state records revealed that 1,354 arrest-related sudden deaths occurred in the United States between January 1, 2006 and December 31, 2013. Analysis of the data begins with a description of basic frequencies.

DESCRIPTION OF ARREST-RELATED DEATH STATISTICS

The most arrest-related sudden deaths (236) occurred in 2006. The fewest deaths (136) occurred in 2012. Figure 1, Total Arrest-Related Sudden Deaths by Year, shows the number of deaths by year over the period of 2006 through 2013. Trend analysis (y = -11.29x + 220.04) indicates that arrest-related sudden deaths decreased, on average, by slightly more than 11 deaths per year. The coefficient and error terms in the trend equation were truncated and rounded to two decimal places.

Of the 1,354 arrest-related sudden deaths, 534 deaths (39.4 percent) followed the application of a TASER ECD. Although the other 820 deaths (60.6 percent) might have involved the use of other force options, they did not involve the use of an ECD, according to available information. The most non-ECD deaths and the most ECD-proximate deaths (156 and 80, respectively) occurred in 2006. The fewest non-ECD deaths (75) were in 2008. The fewest ECD-proximate deaths (56) occurred in 2013. Figure 2, Non-ECD versus ECD-Proximate Arrest-Related Sudden Deaths by Year, shows the number of deaths in each group from 2006 through 2013. Trend analysis indicates that, on average, non-ECD deaths decreased more than 8.1 per year (y = -8.14x + 139.14), and ECD-proximate deaths decreased more than 3.1 per year (y = -3.14x + 80.89) from 2006 through 2013. The coefficient and error terms in the trend line equations were truncated and rounded to two decimal places.

Figure 1. Total Arrest-Related Sudden Deaths by Year

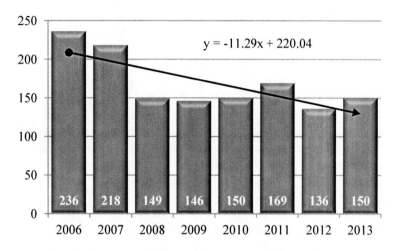

Figure 2. Non-ECD versus ECD-Proximate Arrest-Related Sudden Deaths by Year

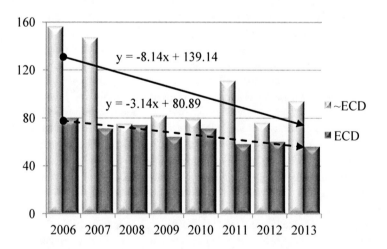

The highest ratio of ECD-proximate deaths to total arrest-related sudden deaths (0.50) was in 2008, while the lowest ratio (0.33) was in 2007. Table 1, Ratio of ECD Arrest-Related Sudden Deaths by Year, shows the numbers of deaths each year (All), the number of deaths that were not associated with the use of a TASER ECD (~ECD), the number of deaths that were proximate to the use of a TASER ECD (ECD), and the ratio of deaths associated with the use of a TASER ECD compared to all arrest-related sudden deaths each year (ECD/All). In no year did ECD-proximate deaths exceed non-ECD deaths, although the non-ECD and ECD-proximate deaths were nearly equal in 2008. The ratios in Table 1 were truncated and rounded to two decimal places.

Table 1. Ratio of ECD Arrest-Related Sudden Deaths by Year

Year	All	~ECD	ECD	ECD/All
2006	236	156	80	0.34
2007	218	147	71	0.33
2008	149	75	74	0.50
2009	146	82	64	0.44
2010	150	79	71	0.47
2011	169	111	58	0.34
2012	136	76	60	0.44
2013	150	94	56	0.37
Total	1,354	820	534	0.39

LOGISTIC REGRESSION ANALYSIS

Two logistic regression (logit) models were constructed. In both models, the use of a TASER ECD (ECD) was set as a dichotomous dependent variable with values of 0 (no) and 1 (yes). Age was set as a continuous variable, with values ranging from 16 to 87, the range of ages of the deceased within the population. Sex was set with dichotomous values of 0 (female) and 1 (male). Race/ethnicity was set with dichotomous variables of 0 (White) and 1 (all other races and ethnicities). The other predictor variables were set with dichotomous values of 0 (the variable was not observed) and 1 (the variable was observed).

In model one, use of an ECD was regressed on the primary tenets of high-risk group theory, age (AGE), cardiovascular disease (CVD), implantable cardioverter defibrillators (ICD), drugs present (DAP), a history of drug abuse (HDA), excited delirium (ExDS), alcohol present (AP), history of chronic alcohol abuse (HCAA), mental illness (MT), and psychotropic medications (PM). Additionally, sex and race/ethnicity were added to the model to determine whether those variables had an effect on the frequency of deaths involving an ECD.

Model two was a more parsimonious model. Only two cases presented with a pacemaker or implantable cardioverter/defibrillator, and both of those cases were diagnosed with cardiovascular disease. One case was a non-ECD death, and one case was an ECD-proximate death. Because it appeared that consideration of the ICD variable could add little to the analysis, the ICD variable was dropped from model two. Additionally, in five cases, medical examiners and coroners did not record mental illness in the autopsy report, but toxicology reports indicated the presence of psychotropic medications. Such medications are not generally consumed for recreational purposes, so it was likely that the deceased was taking them to treat a mental illness. Moreover, mental illness is not observable at autopsy. Toxicology tests can reveal the existence of drugs and medications, but there is no post-mortem test for mental illness. Medical examiners or coroners might have been reticent to document a mental illness in the autopsy report without supporting medical documentation. Additionally, collinearity computations indicate that mental illness and psychotropic medications are collinear (adjusted LR $\chi^2(1) = 100.24$). Therefore, the mental illness and psychotropic medications variables were re-coded to combine them into one mental illness variable (MNTL) for model two. Table 2, Logistic Regression Analysis of Attribute Data, contains the output for the logit models. Appendix D, STATA Regression Model Tables, contains the complete tables for all logit models. Significance was set at $|z| \geq 1.96$.

DEMOGRAPHICS

Age is a tenet of high-risk group theory, but sex and race/ethnicity are not. Nonetheless, data regarding the sex and race/ethnicity factors of arrest-related sudden deaths are included to aid in understanding potential demographic effects on arrest-related sudden deaths and high-risk group theory.

Table 2. Logistic Regression Analysis of Attribute Data

ECD	Model 1			Model 2		
	O.R.	Coef.	z	O.R.	Coef.	z
AGE	0.9828	-0.0174	-1.33	0.9827	-0.1747	-1.43
SEX	3.1898	1.1600	1.77	2.8032	1.0308	1.75
RACE	0.9563	-0.0446	-0.17	1.0463	0.0452	0.18
CVD	0.9703	-0.0301	-0.11	1.0293	0.2890	0.11
ICD	3.2036	1.1643	0.73	-	-	-
DAP	0.5376	-0.6206	-1.92	0.5265	-0.6415	-2.06
HDA	1.2590	0.2303	0.55	1.2110	0.1915	0.47
ExDS	2.5650	0.9419	3.01	2.8145	1.0348	3.37
ETOH	1.0847	0.0813	0.26	1.0537	0.0523	0.17
HCAA	0.2303	-1.4683	-2.43	0.2430	-1.4148	-2.37
MT	9.6608	2.2680	2.81	-	-	-
PMED	0.2008	-1.6054	-1.86	-	-	-
MNTL	-	-	-	1.8665	0.6240	1.43
_CONS	-	-0.2007	-0.23	-	-0.1370	-0.16

Age Analysis

For the 1,054 cases in the sampling frame for which age data are available, the mean age of ECD-proximate deaths is 36.86 years, which is 1.5 years younger than the mean age of 38.36 years for non-ECD deaths. The 95 percent confidence interval (CI) of the differences of the mean ages is 0.13 to 2.87 years. The median age of ECD-proximate deaths is 36, and the median age of non-ECD deaths is 37. The mode for non-ECD deaths is 34 years. The mode for ECD-proximate deaths is 28 years. Age ranges are comparable for both groups. The age range for non-ECD deaths is 68 years (ages 17 to 85). The age range for ECD-proximate deaths is 71 years (ages 16 to 87).

For the sample of 300 cases, the mean age of ECD-proximate deaths is 37.16 years, or 2.67 years younger than the mean age of 39.83 years for non-ECD deaths. The CI of the difference in the sample mean ages is 0.20 to 5.15 years. The difference of 2.67 years is within the CI of 0.13 to 2.87 years for the mean age difference of the population, meaning the difference in ages between the population and the sample is not statistically significant. The median age for ECD-proximate deaths is 37 years, and the median age for non-ECD deaths is 39.5 years. The mode for non-ECD deaths is 41 years. The mode for ECD-proximate deaths is 36 years. The age range for non-ECD deaths is 55 years (ages 19 to 74 years). The age range for ECD-proximate deaths is 71 years (ages 16 to 87 years).

The hypothesis related to age in high-risk group theory is:

H_{A1}: People who suffer an arrest-related sudden death following application of a TASER ECD are younger than those who suffer an arrest-related sudden death absent the use of a TASER ECD.

Concerning the ages in the sampling frame, the observed difference of 1.5 years corresponds to a *t*-statistic of 2.15, a small effect size of 0.13, and a statistically significant probability of 0.03. Concerning the ages in the sample, the observed difference of 2.67 years corresponds to a *t*-statistic of 2.13, a moderate effect size of 0.25, and a statistically significant probability of 0.03. From the t-test analysis, considering the age variable in isolation, it appears that TASER-proximate deaths are about 1.5 to 2.7 years younger, on average, than non-ECD deaths.

Both logit models indicate that ECD-proximate deaths are younger than non-ECD deaths, with *z*-scores of -1.33 for model one and -1.43 for model two; however, neither of the *z*-scores is statistically significant. The significance evident in the *t*-tests disappears in the logit models that control for other predictor variables. Table 3, headed "Age Data for Arrest-Related Sudden Deaths," displays the descriptive and *t*-test statistics for the age data from the population in the sampling frame and from the sample of 300 cases. The logit outputs are set forth in Table 2. Consequently, the observed difference in ages between non-ECD and ECD-proximate deaths in the sample, while holding constant the other predictor variables, is insufficiently large to conclude that the difference is more than a product of sampling error.

The mean ages for all arrest-related sudden deaths, 37.8 years in the population and 38.25 years in the sample, are older than the mean age of 35.7 years in two previous studies of arrest-related deaths (Ho, Heegaard, et al., 2009; Southall, et al, 2008). The mean age of ECD-proximate deaths in the population (36.8 years) and in the sample (37.2 years) are between 0.9 and 2.4 years older than the mean ages of between 34.8

years and 35.9 years in three previous studies of ECD-proximate deaths (Strote, et al., 2005; White, et al., 2013; Williams, 2008).

Table 3. Age Data for Arrest-Related Sudden Deaths

	Population		Sample	
	~ECD	ECD	~ECD	ECD
N	636	418	150	150
Mean	38.36	36.86	39.83	37.16
Median	37	36	39.5	37
Mode	34	29	41	36
Range	17 – 85	16 – 87	19 – 74	16 – 87
IQ Range	29 – 46	29 – 43.75	31 – 47.75	30.25 – 43
SEM	0.45	0.53	0.91	0.86
SD	11.33	10.74	11.16	10.59
< 20	1.4%	2.4%	0.7%	3.3%
20 – 29	24.1%	25.6%	21.3%	20.0%
30 – 39	30.0%	34.0%	28.0%	37.3%
40 – 49	25.8%	26.8%	29.3%	30.0%
50 – 59	15.6%	8.9%	18.0%	6.7%
60 – 69	2.3%	1.7%	2.0%	2.0%
≥70	0.8%	0.7%	0.7%	0.7%
	$df = 1,052, t = 2.15$		$df = 298, t = 2.13$	
	$SE = 0.53, p = 0.03$		$SE = 1.26, p = 0.03$	
	$r = 0.07, d = 0.13$		$r = 0.13, d = 0.25$	

Sex Analysis
Because publicly available sources identified the sex of every deceased, it is possible to analyze sex data for the 1,060 cases in the population. Men constitute the clear majority of arrest-related sudden deaths (94.2 percent). They are 91.6 percent of non-ECD deaths, and 98.1 percent of ECD-proximate deaths. In the sample, males constitute 93.7 percent of all arrest-related sudden deaths, 90.0 percent of non-ECD deaths, and 97.3 percent of ECD-proximate deaths.

The hypothesis related to sex in high-risk group theory is:

H_{A2}: The frequency of a TASER ECD being involved in an arrest-related sudden death is not the same for men and women.

Concerning sex data in the population, the observed difference corresponds to a χ^2-statistic of 19.41, a moderate effect size of 0.25, and a statistically significant probability of less than 0.01. Concerning sex data in the sample, the observed difference corresponds to a χ^2-statistic of 6.80, a small effect size of 0.15, and a statistically significant probability of less than 0.01, which indicates that the difference in sex in the non-ECD and ECD-proximate groups is independent. Table 4, χ^2 Contingency Table for Sex, summarizes the χ^2 calculations for sex data in the sampling frame and the selected sample.

Table 4. χ^2 Contingency Table for Sex

	Sampling Frame			Sample		
	Female	Male	Total	Female	Male	Total
Non-ECD	54	588	642	15	135	150
ECD	8	410	418	4	146	150
Total	62	998	1,060	19	281	300
	$df = 1$, $\chi^2 = 19.41$			$df = 1$, $\chi^2 = 6.80$		
	$p < 0.01$, $\varphi = -0.14$			$p < 0.01$, $\varphi = -0.15$		
				Yate's $\chi^2 = 5.62$		
				Yate's $p = .02$		

The logit models indicate that men are about 2.8 to 3.2 times more likely to be involved in ECD-proximate deaths than are women. However, controlling for the other predictor variables, that difference is statistically insignificant in both models. The z-scores for sex are 1.77 in model one and 1.75 in model two. Consequently, the difference in sex in the observed sample, while holding constant the other predictor variables, is insufficiently large to conclude that the difference is more than a product of sampling error. The logit outputs are reported in Table 2.

The findings of the current study closely reflect the results of previous studies. Males constitute between 93.3 percent and 96.3 percent of all arrest-related deaths in three previous studies (Burch, 2011; Ho, Heegaard, et al., 2009; Southall, et al., 2005). In two previous studies of ECD-proximate deaths (White, et al., 2013; Williams, 2008), males are between 95.8 percent and 97.4 percent of the deaths.

Race/Ethnicity Analysis
Race/ethnicity data are missing for 204 of the 1,060 cases in the population. Since about 19.2 percent of the data are missing, no statistical calculations are made regarding the race/ethnicity of the sampling frame. Information on race/ethnicity is missing from one case in the sample. Whites comprise 41.6 percent (62 cases) of the non-ECD deaths, more than any other race or ethnicity. Blacks, however, have the most ECD-proximate deaths with 69 (46.0 percent). Deaths for Hispanics and other races/ethnicities are consistent across the categories. The hypothesis related to race/ethnicity in high-risk group theory is:

H_{A3}: The frequency of a TASER ECD being involved in an arrest-related sudden death is not the same for Whites, Blacks, Hispanics, and all other races and ethnicities.

Concerning the race/ethnicity data in the sample, the observed difference corresponds to a χ^2-statistic of 1.10, a small effect size of 0.06, and a statistically insignificant probability of 0.78, findings which indicate that the difference in race/ethnicity in the non-ECD and ECD-proximate groups is independent. Table 5, χ^2 Contingency Table for Race/Ethnicity, summarizes the χ^2 calculations for race/ethnicity data in the sample. In the logit models, race/ethnicity is coded as a dichotomous variable, White (0) and all other races and ethnicities (1). The z-scores in the logit models were -0.17 in model one and 0.18 in model two, indicating that the difference in race/ethnicity in the observed sample, while holding constant the other predictor variables, is insufficiently large to conclude that the difference is more than a product of sampling error. The logit outputs are contained in Table 2.

Table 5. χ^2 Contingency Table for Race/Ethnicity

	Black	White	Hispanic	Other	Total
Non-ECD	60	62	23	4	149
ECD	69	56	22	3	150
Total	129	118	45	7	299

$df = 3$, $\chi^2 = 1.10$, $p = 0.78$, Cramér's $V = 0.06$
Yate's $\chi^2 = 0.69$, Yate's $p = .88$

CARDIOVASCULAR DISEASE ANALYSIS

The second most frequently occurring variable in the sample is cardio-vascular disease. Of the sample of 300, medical examiners and coroners report cardiovascular disease in 164 (54.7 percent). Cardiovascular disease is more prevalent in the non-ECD group (86 cases) than in the ECD-proximate group (78 cases). The mean age at time of death for all cases with cardiovascular disease is 41.0 years. For non-ECD deaths, the mean age is 42.6 years. For ECD-proximate deaths, the mean age is 39.3 years.

The hypothesis related to cardiovascular disease in high-risk group theory is:

H_{A4}:   The frequency of people with cardiovascular diseases suffering arrest-related sudden death is not the same for TASER ECD-proximate deaths and non-ECD deaths.

Concerning cardiovascular disease data in the sample, the observed difference corresponds to a χ^2-statistic of 0.86, a small effect size of 0.05, and a statistically insignificant probability of 0.35, which indicates that the difference in cardiovascular disease in the non-ECD and ECD-proximate groups is independent. Table 6, χ^2 Contingency Table for Cardiovascular Disease, summarizes the χ^2 calculations for cardiovascular disease data in the sample. In the logit models, the z-scores range from -0.11 in model one to 0.11 in model two, indicating that the difference in cardiovascular disease in the observed sample, while holding constant the other predictor variables, is insufficiently large to conclude that the difference is more than a product of sampling error. The logit outputs are set forth in Table 2.

Table 6. χ^2 Contingency Table for Cardiovascular Disease

	No	Yes	Total
Non-ECD	64	86	150
ECD	72	78	150
Total	136	164	300

$$df = 1, \chi^2 = 0.86$$
$$p = 0.35, \varphi = 0.05$$

PACEMAKERS AND ICDS ANALYSIS

Autopsy reports document only two cases in the sample with a pacemaker or ICD. One case is a non-ECD death of a 74-year-old male. The other case is an ECD-proximate death of a 66-year-old male. Insufficient data exists for χ^2 statistical analysis of the H_{A5} hypothesis. Consequently, there is no contingency table for this variable. Logit model one assigns the ICD variable a z-score of 0.73, indicating that the observed difference is not statistically significant. The logit outputs are reported in Table 2.

DRUGS ANALYSIS

The presence of drugs is the most frequently occurring variable in the study. Toxicology reports demonstrate that 219 of the 300 cases in the study (73.0 percent) have drugs in their systems at autopsy. More non-ECD cases than ECD-proximate cases present with drugs, 115 to 104, respectively. The reports document 14 women with drugs in their systems. Three of those 14 women (24.1 percent) are ECD-proximate deaths. Toxicology reports document 205 men with drugs in their systems. Of those 205 men, 49.3 percent (101) are ECD-proximate deaths. Cocaine is present in the most cases (140), followed by amphetamines (57) and marijuana (51). Table 25, Types of Drugs Present, details the type of drugs present in the toxicology reports of the cases in the sample. Because some cases present with more than one type of drug, the numbers add to more than 219.

The hypothesis related to using drugs in high-risk group theory is:

H_{A6}: The frequency of people currently using drugs suffering arrest-related sudden death is not the same for TASER ECD-proximate deaths and non-ECD deaths.

Concerning drug data in the sample, the observed difference between non-ECD and ECD-proximate deaths corresponds to a χ^2-statistic of 2.05, a small effect size of 0.08, and a statistically insignificant probability of 0.15, which indicates that the difference in drugs present in the non-ECD and ECD-proximate groups is independent. Table 7, χ^2 Contingency Table for Drugs Present, summarizes the χ^2 calculations for drugs data in the sample.

Table 7. χ^2 Contingency Table for Drugs Present

	No	Yes	Total
Non-ECD	35	115	150
ECD	46	104	150
Total	81	219	300

$$df = 1, \chi^2 = 2.05$$
$$p = 0.15, \varphi = 0.08$$

In logit model one, which considers the primary variables of high-risk group theory, the z-score for drugs is -1.92, indicating that the difference in drugs in the observed sample, while holding constant the other predictor variables, is insufficiently large to conclude that the difference is more than a product of sampling error. However, in model two, which excludes the ICD variable and collapses the mental illness and psychotropic medications variables, the z-score is -2.06, indicating that the difference in drugs in the observed sample, while holding constant the other predictor variables, is sufficiently large to conclude that the difference is more than sampling error. Additionally, a z-score of -2.06 indicates that drugs are more likely to be involved in non-ECD deaths than in ECD-proximate deaths. Odds ratios in models one and two (truncated and rounded to two decimal places) are 0.54 and 0.53, respectively, indicating that drugs are about 1.9 times more likely to be involved in non-ECD deaths than in ECD-proximate deaths. The logit outputs are reported in Table 2.

Sufficient information on the use of drugs exists to allow for χ^2 analysis on supplemental hypotheses for the presence of amphetamines, cocaine, marijuana, opiates, and PCP. Because there is only one case involving the LSD variable, insufficient data points exist to formulate a supplemental hypothesis regarding the use of LSD.

Amphetamine Analysis
Amphetamines are the second most prevalent drug present in toxicology reports. Fifty-seven cases present with amphetamines during autopsy, 29 non-ECD deaths and 28 ECD-proximate deaths. Five amphetamine cases are females. Four of those five are non-ECD cases, and one is an ECD-proximate case. Males comprise 52 amphetamine cases. Twenty-five of the 52 cases are non-ECD cases, and 27 were ECD-proximate deaths. The mean age of the non-ECD amphetamine deaths

is 39.1 years. The mean age of the ECD-proximate amphetamine deaths is 35.1 years.

The hypotheses related to amphetamines use in high-risk group theory is:

$H_{A6.1}$: The frequency of people currently using amphetamines suffering arrest-related sudden death is not the same for TASER ECD-proximate deaths and non-ECD deaths.

Concerning use of amphetamines in the sample, the observed difference corresponds to a χ^2-statistic of 0.02, a small effect size of 0.01, and a statistically insignificant probability of 0.88, which indicates that the difference in amphetamines present in the non-ECD and ECD-proximate groups is independent. Table 8, χ^2 Contingency Table for Amphetamines Present, summarizes the χ^2 calculations for amphetamine use data in the sample.

Table 8. χ^2 Contingency Table for Amphetamines Present

	No	Yes	Total
Non-ECD	121	29	150
ECD	122	28	150
Total	243	57	300
	$df = 1, \chi^2 = 0.02$		
	$p = 0.88, \varphi = 0.01$		

Cocaine Analysis
Cocaine is the most prevalent drug present in toxicology reports. Of the 300 cases in the sample, 140 cases (77 non-ECD deaths and 63 ECD-proximate deaths) present with cocaine at autopsy. Nine cocaine cases are females. Seven of those nine cases are non-ECD cases, and two cases are ECD-proximate deaths. Males comprise 131 cocaine cases. Of those 131 cases, 70 are non-ECD cases, and 61 are ECD-proximate deaths. The mean age of non-ECD cocaine deaths is 37.7 years. The mean age of ECD-proximate cocaine deaths is 36.4 years.

The hypotheses related to cocaine use in high-risk group theory is:

$H_{A6.2}$: The frequency of people currently using cocaine suffering arrest-related sudden death is not the same for TASER ECD-proximate deaths and non-ECD deaths.

Concerning the cocaine data in the sample, the observed difference corresponds to a χ^2-statistic of 2.63, a small effect size of 0.09, and a statistically insignificant probability of 0.11, which indicates that the difference in cocaine present in the non-ECD and ECD-proximate groups is independent. Table 9, χ^2 Contingency Table for Cocaine Present, summarizes the χ^2 calculations for cocaine use data in the sample.

Table 9. χ^2 Contingency Table for Cocaine Present

	No	Yes	Total
Non-ECD	73	77	150
ECD	87	63	150
Total	160	140	300

$$df = 1, \chi^2 = 2.63$$
$$p = 0.11, \varphi = 0.09$$

LSD Analysis
A single case, a 19-year old white male, presents with LSD present at autopsy. The case is a non-ECD death. Insufficient data exist for any χ^2 calculations of the LSD present variable, so there is no contingency table for this variable.

Marijuana Analysis
Fifty-one cases present with marijuana during autopsy, 25 are non-ECD deaths, and 26 are ECD-proximate deaths. One case, a non-ECD death, is female. Males comprise the other 50 marijuana cases. Twenty-four of the 50 cases are non-ECD deaths, and 26 cases are ECD-proximate deaths. The mean age of the non-ECD marijuana deaths is 35.4 years. The mean age of the ECD-proximate marijuana deaths is 31.5 years.

The hypotheses related to marijuana use in high-risk group theory is:

$H_{A6.3}$: The frequency of people currently using marijuana suffering arrest-related sudden death is not the same for TASER ECD-proximate deaths and non-ECD deaths.

Concerning marijuana data in the sample, the observed difference corresponds to a χ^2-statistic of 0.02, a small effect size of -0.01, and a statistically insignificant probability of 0.88, which indicates that the difference in marijuana present in the non-ECD and ECD-proximate groups is independent. Table 10, χ^2 Contingency Table for Marijuana Present, summarizes the χ^2 calculations for marijuana use data in the sample.

Table 10. χ^2 Contingency Table for Marijuana Present

	No	Yes	Total
Non-ECD	125	25	150
ECD	124	26	150
Total	249	51	300

$$df = 1, \chi^2 = 0.02$$
$$p = 0.88, \varphi = -0.01$$

Opiates Analysis
Thirty-five cases present with opiates during autopsy, 21 are non-ECD deaths, and 14 are ECD-proximate deaths. Three cases, all non-ECD deaths, are female. Males comprise 32 opiate cases. Nineteen of the 32 cases are non-ECD deaths, and 13 are ECD-proximate deaths. The mean age of the non-ECD opiate deaths is 42.4 years. The mean age of the ECD-proximate opiate deaths is 38.2 years.

The hypothesis related to opiates use in high-risk group theory is:

$H_{A6.4}$: The frequency of people currently using opiates suffering arrest-related sudden death is not the same for TASER ECD-proximate deaths and non-ECD deaths.

Concerning opiates data in the sample, the observed difference corresponds to a χ^2-statistic of 2.62, a small effect size of 0.09, and a statistically insignificant probability of 0.11, which indicates that the difference in opiates present in the non-ECD and ECD-proximate groups is independent. Table 11, χ^2 Contingency Table for Opiates Present, summarizes the χ^2 calculations for opiate use data in the sample.

Table 11. χ^2 Contingency Table for Opiates Present

	No	Yes	Total
Non-ECD	128	22	150
ECD	137	13	150
Total	265	35	300

$$df = 1, \chi^2 = 2.62$$
$$p = 0.11, \varphi = 0.09$$

PCP Analysis

Thirteen cases present with PCP during autopsy, four are non-ECD deaths, and nine are ECD-proximate deaths. One case, a non-ECD death, is female. Males comprise the other 12 opiate cases. Three of those 12 cases are non-ECD cases, and nine are ECD-proximate deaths. The mean age of the non-ECD PCP deaths is 30.0 years. The mean age of the ECD-proximate PCP deaths is 33.1 years.

The hypothesis related to PCP use in high-risk group theory is:

$H_{A6.5}$: The frequency of people currently using PCP suffering arrest-related sudden death is not the same for TASER ECD-proximate deaths and non-ECD deaths.

Concerning PCP data in the sample, the observed difference corresponds to a χ^2-statistic of 2.01, a small effect size of -0.08, and a statistically insignificant probability of 0.16, which indicates that the difference in PCP present in the non-ECD and ECD-proximate groups is independent. Table 12, χ^2 Contingency Table for PCP Present, summarizes the χ^2 calculations for PCP use data in the sample.

Table 12. χ^2 Contingency Table for PCP Present

	No	Yes	Total
Non-ECD	146	4	150
ECD	141	9	150
Total	287	13	300

$$df = 1, \chi^2 = 2.01$$
$$p = 0.16, \varphi = -0.08$$
$$\text{Yate's } \chi^2 = 1.29$$
$$\text{Yate's } p = .26$$

History of Drug Abuse Analysis

In 35 cases, medical examiners or coroners refer to the deceased's history of abusing drugs. In 32 cases, they make this reference concurrent with a notation of the presence of drugs in the body of the deceased. In three cases, however, the autopsy reveals no drugs in the system of the deceased. Of the 35 reported cases of history of drug abuse, four are female. All four of those cases are non-ECD deaths. Males comprise 31 history of drug abuse cases. Twelve of the 31 cases are non-ECD cases, and 19 are ECD-proximate deaths. The mean age of the non-ECD history of drug abuse deaths is 38.6 years. The mean age of the ECD-proximate history of drug abuse deaths is 34.2 years.

The hypothesis related to history of drug abuse in high-risk group theory is:

H_{A7}: The frequency of people with a history of drug abuse suffering arrest-related sudden death is not the same for TASER ECD-proximate deaths and non-ECD deaths.

Concerning history of drug abuse in the sample, the observed difference corresponds to a χ^2-statistic of 0.81, a small effect size of -0.03, and a statistically insignificant probability of 0.37, which indicates that the difference in history of drug abuse in the non-ECD and ECD-proximate groups is independent. Table 13, χ^2 Contingency Table for History of Drug Abuse, summarizes the χ^2 calculations for history of drug abuse data in the sample.

The z-scores in logit model one and model two are 0.55 and 0.47, respectively, indicating that the difference in history of drug abuse in the observed sample, while holding constant the other predictor variables, is insufficiently large to conclude that the difference is more than a product of sampling error. The logit outputs are reported in Table 2.

Table 13. χ^2 Contingency Table for History of Drug Abuse

	No	Yes	Total
Non-ECD	134	16	150
ECD	131	19	150
Total	265	35	300
	$df = 1, \chi^2 = 0.81$		
	$p = 0.37, \varphi = -0.03$		

EXCITED DELIRIUM ANALYSIS

Medical examiners and coroners classify 77 cases (25.7 percent) as ExDS. Of those cases, only one is female. That ECD-proximate case involves a 35-year-old female. Of the 76 ExDS cases involving men, 23 cases are non-ECD deaths, and 53 cases are ECD-proximate deaths. The mean age of the non-ECD deaths is 36.5 years. The mean age of the ECD-proximate deaths is 35.3 years.

In five of the ExDS cases medical examiners or coroners refer to neither mental illness nor presence of drugs. In six cases, the deceased are mentally ill. In 60 cases, the deceased have drugs in their systems at autopsy. In six cases, the deceased are both mentally ill and have drugs in their systems.

The hypothesis related to ExDS in high-risk group theory is:

H_{A8}: The frequency of people exhibiting symptoms of ExDS suffering arrest-related sudden death is not the same for TASER ECD-proximate deaths and non-ECD deaths.

Concerning ExDS data in the sample, the observed difference corresponds to a χ^2-statistic of 16.79, a moderate effect size of 0.24, and a statistically significant probability of less than 0.01, which indicates that the difference in ExDS in the non-ECD and ECD-proximate groups is dependent. Table 14, χ^2 Contingency Table for Excited Delirium, summarizes the χ^2 calculations for ExDS data in the sample.

Table 14. χ^2 Contingency Table for Excited Delirium

	No	Yes	Total
Non-ECD	127	23	150
ECD	96	54	150
Total	223	77	300
		$df = 1, \chi^2 = 16.79$	
		$p < 0.01, \varphi = -0.24$	

For the ExDS variable, the logit models calculate statistically significant z-scores ranging of from 3.01 in model one to 3.57 in model two, indicating that the difference in ExDS in the observed sample, while holding constant the other predictor variables, is sufficiently large to conclude that the difference is more than sampling error. Therefore, evidence supports that ECD-proximate deaths involving ExDS occur more frequently than non-ECD deaths involving ExDS. The logit outputs are reported in Table 2.

ALCOHOL ANALYSIS

In 59 cases (19.7 percent), toxicology reports reveal the presence of alcohol at autopsy. Of those 59 cases, 30 cases are non-ECD deaths, and 29 cases are ECD-proximate deaths. Only one case, a non-ECD death, involves a female, who is 34 years of age. Of the 58 cases involving males, 29 are non-ECD deaths, and 29 are ECD-proximate deaths. The mean age of the non-ECD deaths is 41.3 years. The mean age of the ECD-proximate deaths is 36.6 years. Of the 59 alcohol cases, 44 have drugs in their systems at autopsy, seven have a history of chronic alcohol abuse, one is mentally ill, and three are mentally ill and have drugs in their systems.

The hypothesiss related to alcohol present in high-risk group theory is:

H_{A9}: The frequency of people intoxicated from alcohol suffering arrest-related sudden death is not the same for TASER ECD-proximate deaths and non-ECD deaths.

Concerning alcohol data in the sample, the observed difference corresponds to a χ^2-statistic of 0.02, a small effect size of 0.01, and a statistically insignificant probability of 0.89, which indicates that the difference in alcohol in the non-ECD and ECD-proximate groups is independent. Table 15, χ^2 Contingency Table for Alcohol Present, summarizes the χ^2 calculations for alcohol present data in the sample.

Table 15. χ^2 Contingency Table for Alcohol Present

	No	Yes	Total
Non-ECD	120	30	150
ECD	121	29	150
Total	241	59	300
	$df = 1, \chi^2 = 0.02$		
	$p = 0.89, \varphi = 0.01$		

For the alcohol variable, the logit models calculate statistically insignificant z-scores of 0.17 to 0.52, indicating that the difference in alcohol in the observed sample, while holding constant the other predictor variables, is insufficiently large to conclude that the difference is more than a product of sampling error. The logit outputs are set forth in Table 2.

Chronic Alcohol Abuse Analysis

In 22 cases, or 7.3 percent, medical examiners or coroners report a history of chronic alcohol abuse. Of those 22 cases, 18 cases are non-ECD deaths, and four cases are ECD-proximate deaths. In the two cases involving females, one case is a non-ECD death, and one case is an ECD-proximate death. Of the 20 cases involving males, 17 cases are non-ECD deaths, and three cases are ECD-proximate deaths. The mean age of the non-ECD deaths is 47.8 years. The mean age of the ECD-proximate deaths is 39.0 years.

The hypothesis related to chronic alcohol abuse in high-risk group theory is:

H_{A10}: The frequency of people with a history of chronic alcohol abuse suffering arrest-related sudden death is not the same for TASER ECD-proximate deaths and non-ECD deaths.

Concerning chronic alcohol abuse in the sample, the observed difference corresponds to a χ^2-statistic of 9.61, a small effect size of 0.18, and a statistically significant probability of less than 0.01, which indicates that the difference in chronic alcohol abuse in the non-ECD and ECD-proximate groups is dependent. Table 16, χ^2 Contingency Table for Chronic Alcohol Abuse, summarizes the χ^2 calculations for chronic alcohol abuse data in the sample.

Table 16. χ^2 Contingency Table for Chronic Alcohol Abuse

	No	Yes	Total
Non-ECD	132	18	150
ECD	146	4	150
Total	278	22	300

$$df = 1, \chi^2 = 9.61$$
$$p < 0.01, \varphi = 0.18$$
$$\text{Yate's } \chi^2 = 8.29$$
$$\text{Yate's } p < 0.01$$

For the chronic alcohol abuse variable, both logit models calculate statistically significant z-scores, -2.43 in model one and -2.28 in model two, indicating that the difference in history of chronic alcohol abuse in the observed sample, while holding constant the other predictor variables, is sufficiently large to conclude that the difference is more than sampling error. Therefore, evidence supports that ECD-proximate deaths involving chronic alcohol abuse occur less frequently than non-ECD deaths involving chronic alcohol abuse. The logit outputs are displayed in Table 2.

MENTAL ILLNESS ANALYSIS

In 29 cases, or 9.7 percent, medical examiners or coroners report that the deceased is mentally ill or has a history of mental illness. Of those 29 cases, five cases are non-ECD deaths, and 24 cases are ECD-proximate deaths. Two cases involve females, both of which are ECD-proximate deaths. Of the 27 cases involving males, five are non-ECD cases, and 22 are ECD-proximate cases. The mean age of the non-ECD deaths is 41.2 years. The mean age of the ECD-proximate deaths is 37.4 years. Of the 29 mental illness cases, toxicology reports indicate that 13 are taking medications for the illness. Eleven of the deceased have ExDS, seven present with drugs in their systems at autopsy, and three have alcohol in their systems.

The hypothesis related to mental illness in high-risk group theory is:

H_{A11}: The frequency of people with mental illness suffering arrest-related sudden death is not the same for TASER ECD-proximate deaths and non-ECD deaths.

Concerning mental illness in the sample, the observed difference corresponds to a χ^2-statistic of 13.78, a moderate effect size of 0.21, and a statistically significant probability of less than 0.01, which indicates that the difference in mental illness in the non-ECD and ECD-proximate groups is dependent. Table 16, χ^2 Contingency Table for Mental Illness, summarizes the χ^2 calculations for mental illness data in the sample.

The logit models show some interesting results. Model one, which analyzes mental illness and psychotropic medications as unique variables, calculates a z-score of 2.81 for the mental illness variable. That z-score is statistically significant, indicating that the difference in mental illness in the observed sample, while holding constant the other predictor variables, is sufficiently large to conclude that the difference is more than sampling error. However, the significance disappears when combining the mental illness and psychotropic medications variables in model two. The z-score for the combined mental illness variable is 1.43, indicating that the difference in mental illness in the observed sample, while holding constant the other predictor variables, is insufficiently large to conclude that the difference is more than a product of sampling error. The logit outputs are reported in Table 2.

Table 17. χ^2 Contingency Table for Mental Illness

	No	Yes	Total
Non-ECD	145	5	150
ECD	126	24	150
Total	271	29	300

$$df = 1, \chi^2 = 13.78$$
$$p < 0.01, \varphi = 0.21$$

Psychotropic Medications Analysis
In 18 cases, toxicology reports indicate the presence of psychotropic medications. In five of those cases, medical examiners or coroners record no corresponding mental illness. One case, an ECD-proximate death, involves a 56-year-old female. Of the 17 cases involving males, eight cases are non-ECD deaths, and nine cases are ECD-proximate deaths. Of the 18 medication cases, seven cases have cardiovascular disease, five have drugs in their systems, and four have ExDS.

The hypothesis related to psychotropic medications in high-risk group theory is:

H_{A12}:   The frequency of people taking psychotropic medications suffering arrest-related sudden death is not the same for TASER ECD-proximate deaths and non-ECD deaths.

Concerning psychotropic medications in the sample, the observed difference corresponds to a χ^2-statistic of 0.24, a statistically insignificant probability of 0.63, and a small effect size of 0.03, which indicates that the difference in psychotropic medications in the non-ECD and ECD-proximate groups is independent. Table 18, χ^2 Contingency Table for Psychotropic Medications, summarizes the χ^2 calculations for psychotropic medication data in the sample. Logit model one, the only model to analyze the psychotropic medications variable, calculates a z-

score of -1.86, indicating that the difference in psychotropic medications in the observed sample, while holding constant the other predictor
variables, is insufficiently large to conclude that the difference is more
than a product of sampling error. The logit outputs are contained in
Table 2.

Table 18. χ^2 Contingency Table for Psychotropic Medications

	No	Yes	Total
Non-ECD	142	8	150
ECD	140	10	150
Total	282	18	300
	$df = 1, \chi^2 = 0.24$		
	$p = 0.63, \varphi = 0.03$		

QUALITATIVE COMPARATIVE ANALYSIS

Bivariate contingency table analysis, such as χ^2 calculations, represents
a common method of examining the distribution of two categorical
variables, and it is often used in social science and criminal justice research. Multivariate analysis, such as logit models, can extend an examination to multiple categorical variables and the analysis of main and
interaction effects among them (Meithe, Hart, and Regoeczi, 2008).
QCA shares with these conventional quantitative methods a common
assumption, that the possibility of a variable's impact is consistent
across various contexts. However, QCA also views cases as complex
configurations of attributes, which permits a presumption of causal
complexity.

In this model, the use of a TASER ECD (ECD) is set as the outcome variable. The other variables, cardiovascular disease (CVD),
drugs present (DAP), excited delirium syndrome (ExDS), alcohol present (ETOH), and the combined variable mental illness plus psychotropic medications (MNIL), are set as possible causal conditions. Five
variables of high-risk group theory are not included in the csQCA analysis. The pacemakers and ICD variable has only two cases and, thus,
lacks sufficient data points for consideration. History of drug abuse
and history of chronic alcohol abuse are excluded in favor of the current variables of drugs present and alcohol present. Excluding those
three conditions helps to preserve the parsimony of the model and to
avoid creating problems of limited diversity and individualized expla-

nations. The multiple applications and pregnancy variables of high-risk group theory are not included in the study.

Of the 32 causal condition configurations possible from five dichotomous variables, 24 configurations emerge from the data. Table 19, csQCA Case Configurations by Cell Frequency, displays a truth table listing causal condition configurations of the 300 cases in the sample arranged by most frequently to least frequently occurring configurations. **The most frequent configuration is cardiovascular disease and drugs.** That combination, containing 65 cases and noted in Boolean terms as CVD*DAP*exds*etoh*mnil (capital letters indicating the presence of a variable and lower case letters indicating the absence of the variable), has a consistency of 0.4462, which means that **44.62 percent of the 65 cases in the configuration are ECD-proximate deaths**.

A consistency score of one means that all of the cases in that configuration are ECD-proximate deaths. A consistency score of zero means that all of the cases in that configuration are non-ECD deaths. *Consistency scores between zero and one indicate a conflicting configuration, meaning the configuration is uniquely associated neither with ECD-proximate deaths nor with non-ECD deaths.* Of the 24 configurations in the truth table, 17 are conflicting, and seven have a consistency score of one. None of the configurations has a consistency score of zero.

A prime implicant is a logical, not mathematical or statistical, reduction of the conditions in a case configuration to identify conditions necessary and sufficient to produce an outcome. For example, assume a number of cases that contain condition A, condition B, condition C, and condition D all produce a specific outcome. In Boolean terms, that configuration appears as A*B*C*D → O. Next, assume another set of cases that contain condition A, condition B, and condition C, but not condition D produces the same outcome. In Boolean terms, that configuration appears as A*B*C*d → O. Looking at the two Boolean equations, one can see that the outcome exists whenever conditions A, B, and C exist together, regardless of whether condition D exists, which renders condition D irrelevant to the outcome. Therefore, the causal condition equation can be reduced to A*B*C → O.

Table 19. csQCA Case Configurations by Cell Frequency

CVD	DAP	ExDS	ETOH	MNIL	Freq.	Cons.
1	1	0	0	0	65	0.4462
0	1	0	0	0	52	0.3462
1	0	0	0	0	29	0.4483
0	1	1	0	0	28	0.6071
1	1	0	1	0	20	0.3000
1	1	1	0	0	19	0.6316
0	0	0	0	0	14	0.5714
0	1	0	1	0	10	0.5000
0	1	1	1	0	9	0.7778
0	0	0	0	1	9	0.7778
1	0	0	1	0	9	0.2222
1	0	0	0	1	6	0.6667
1	1	1	1	0	4	1.0000
1	1	0	0	1	4	0.2500
0	1	1	0	1	3	0.6667
0	1	0	1	1	3	0.3333
0	0	1	0	1	3	1.0000
0	0	1	0	0	3	0.6667
1	1	1	0	1	2	1.0000
1	0	1	0	1	2	1.0000
1	0	1	0	0	2	0.5000
0	0	0	1	0	2	1.0000
1	1	1	1	1	1	1.0000
1	0	1	1	1	1	1.0000

The entire sequence of causal configurations can be examined and reduced until only conditions necessary and sufficient to produce the outcome appear in the equation. Of course, the equation can contain more than one set of prime implicants. Assume that other sets of conditions reduce to A*b*D → O. This equation means that condition A and condition D must exist together, but condition B must be absent to produce the outcome. Now two prime implicants indicate two paths to the same outcome: A*B*C or A*b*D. The Boolean notation for the prime implicants equation becomes A*B*C + A*b*D → O. This logical reduction can only occur, however, when all configurations in the truth table are free of conflicting configurations.

Attempts were made to resolve conflicting configurations and establish all configurations with consistencies of 0 or 1 using two of the steps suggested by Rihoux and De Meur (2009): (1) adding conditions to the model one at a time and re-analyzing, and (2) removing conditions from the model and replacing them with other conditions. Adding the pacemaker and ICD variable, history of drug abuse, and history of chronic alcohol abuse one at a time and in combinations did not remove all conflicting configurations, but it added to the complexity of the truth table. Removing the drugs present condition and replacing it with the six constituent drugs (amphetamine, cocaine, LSD, marijuana, opiates, and PCP) did not resolve all conflicting conditions. Expanding the mental illness and psychotropic medication variables back into unique variables did not resolve the conflicts, and neither did collapsing the alcohol present and history of chronic alcohol abuse variables. Thus, *the truth table was not fit for logical minimization.* Several rows always contained conflicting configurations, and it was not possible to deduce prime implicants, those configurations necessary and sufficient to explain the outcome. *The inability to reduce the truth table configurations to any prime implicant provides evidence that the causal conditions differ little between non-ECD deaths and ECD-proximate deaths.*

The truth table illustrates the problem of analyzing complex conditions through χ^2 analysis. Of the 24 configurations that emerge from the data, only five configurations totaling 95 cases contain a single high-risk group theory variable. Four of the five single condition configurations, DAP (52 cases), CVD (29 cases), MNIL (nine cases) and ExDS (three cases), result in conflicting configurations. One single condition configuration, ETOH (two cases), results in a consistency of one, meaning all included cases are ECD-proximate deaths. One configuration of 14 cases exhibits none of the variables of high-risk group theory. That configuration is conflicting.

The remaining 19 configurations, which consist of 205 of the 300 cases, contain two or more conditions. Seven of those 19 configurations had consistencies of one. However, none of those configurations had more than four cases, which means the configurations could be an artifact of limited diversity and individualization of explanations. One configuration containing only one case reflects all five conditions.

Problems of greater interpretative complexity, increased heterogeneity, and small cell frequency sizes often limit applications of csQCA to fewer than 100 case configurations (Meithe, et al., 2008). A case sample of 300, such as in this study, tends to preclude the possibility of non-conflicting consistencies within the truth table. Nevertheless, csQCA is still useful for examining the effects of various variables. A basic starting point in csQCA is an examination of central tendencies and variability in the data that can reveal patterns of clustering and variability among the case configurations. Simple inspection of truth table case configurations can reveal patterns referred to as *situational clustering*. This visual inspection provides evidence of low frequency configurations that can adversely affect regression analysis because of the possible role of low frequency configurations as outliers. Minimum frequency rules, such as deleting configurations with frequency counts less than ten, can reduce the influence of low frequency configurations on substantive conclusions (Meithe, et al., 2008; Ragin 1987).

Recognition of uneven distribution of cell frequencies is important because of the potential for adverse impact of small cell frequencies and multicollinearity on estimating effects within logistic regression analyses. Application of minimum cell frequency rules prevents estimating a saturated model of interactions, but eliminating low-frequency configurations with counts less than ten might generate more stable estimates of net effects (Meithe, et al., 2008; Ragin 1987).

To examine the effects of the variables associated with high-risk group theory, the truth table was first rearranged to rank case configurations according to the relative risks of an arrest-related sudden death being associated with the use of a TASER ECD (i.e. the highest consistency score to the lowest). Next, case configurations with a frequency cell count less than ten were excluded from consideration. The resulting model consisting of eight configurations is shown in Table 19, csQCA Case Configuration by Relative Consistency.

Only three case configurations have consistency scores higher than 0.5000, which means that only those three significant configurations occur more frequently in ECD-proximate deaths than they occur in non-ECD deaths. One configuration has a score of 0.5000, meaning that configuration occurs equally in ECD-proximate and in non-ECD deaths. The other four configurations, which comprise the two highest frequency counts, have consistency scores lower than 0.5000, which means those configurations occur more frequently in non-ECD deaths than they occur in ECD-proximate deaths.

DAP appears in six configurations, CVD appears in four configurations, and ExDS and ETOH each appear in two configurations. MNIL does not appear in any of the eight substantial configurations. The two case configurations that occur most frequently in ECD-proximate deaths (about 63.2 percent and 60.7 percent, respectively) are CVD*DAP*ExDS*etoh*mnil and cvd*DAP*ExDS*etoh*mnil. The two configurations that occur least frequently in ECD-proximate cases are cvd*DAP*exds*etoh*mnil and CVD*DAP*exds*ETOH* mnil (about 34.6 percent and 30.0 percent, respectively).

A simple visual inspection of the data in Table 19 clearly reveals that the two configurations containing ExDS are the only configurations containing a variable of high-risk group theory that occur more frequently in ECD-proximate deaths than in non-ECD deaths. None of the configurations that occur more frequently in non-ECD deaths contains ExDS. The only other configuration more likely to appear in ECD-proximate deaths than in non-ECD deaths contains none of the variables associated with high-risk group theory.

Although the two substantial case configurations most likely to occur in ECD-proximate deaths also contain the drugs present variable, three of the other four case configurations in the model containing drugs are more likely to occur in non-ECD deaths. One drugs present configuration is split equally between non-ECD and ECD-proximate deaths. It is only when drugs interact with ExDS does the configuration become more likely to occur in ECD-proximate deaths.

The case configuration most frequently associated with an ECD-proximate death also contains the cardiovascular disease variable. However, alone, the cardiovascular disease variable occurs more frequently in non-ECD deaths. Even when interacting with the drugs variable alone or with the drugs and alcohol variables together, cardiovascular disease occurs more frequently in non-ECD deaths. It is only when it interacts with ExDS does cardiovascular disease occur more frequently in ECD-proximate deaths.

Only two configurations contain the alcohol variable, and it does not exist alone as a significant configuration. Alcohol and drugs together are equally likely to be involved in non-ECD deaths as they are to be involved in ECD-proximate deaths. When interacting with drugs and cardiovascular disease, the configuration becomes the least frequent ECD-proximate death configuration.

SUMMARY

Results of the statistical analysis of arrest-related sudden death data are summarized as following:

- Examined independently with a Student's *t*-test, people in the sample who suffer an arrest-related sudden death following application of a TASER ECD are approximately 2.67 years younger than those people who suffer an arrest-related sudden death absent the use of a TASER ECD, that difference being statistically significant ($df = 298$, $t = 2.13$, $p = 0.03$). However, in the logit models, when controlling for other predictive variables, the difference in ages between the groups is insufficiently large to establish statistical significance ($z = -1.33$ and $z = -1.43$).
- Sex data from the sample indicates that arrest-related sudden deaths following application of a TASER ECD more frequently involve males than females, the effect size is small ($df = 1$, $\chi^2 = 6.80$, $p < 0.01$, $\varphi = 0.15$). In the logit models, the difference in sex in the sample is insufficiently large to establish statistical significance ($z = 1.77$ and $z = 1.75$).
- Examined by χ^2 analysis using four categorical designations for race, the frequency of an arrest-related sudden death following application of a TASER ECD compared to deaths not involving an ECD is the same for Whites, Blacks, Hispanics, and other races/ethnicities ($df = 3$, $\chi^2 = 1.10$, $p = 0.78$, Cramér's $V = 0.06$). Designated as a dichotomous variable of White = 0 and all other races/ethnicities = 1 for the logit models, the difference in race is statistically insignificant in both models ($z = -0.17$ and $z = 0.18$).
- Analyzed through χ^2, the difference in arrest-related sudden deaths following application of a TASER ECD compared to deaths not involving an ECD is statistically insignificant for

people with cardiovascular diseases ($df = 1$, $\chi^2 = 0.86$, $p = 0.35$, $\varphi = 0.05$). In the logit models, the difference observed in cardiovascular disease is insufficiently large to establish statistical significance ($z = -0.26$ and $z = -0.11$).

- Insufficient data exist to analyze the significance of the pacemakers and ICD variable.

- When calculated with χ^2, the difference in frequencies between arrest-related sudden deaths involving drugs following application of TASER ECDs compared to deaths not involving an ECD is insufficiently large to establish statistical significance ($df = 1$, $\chi^2 = 2.05$, $p = 0.15$, $\varphi = 0.08$). That relationship holds true for individual analyses of amphetamine ($df = 1$, $\chi^2 = 0.02$, $p = 0.88$, $\varphi = 0.01$), cocaine ($df = 1$, $\chi^2 = 2.63$, $p = 0.11$, $\varphi = 0.09$), marijuana ($df = 1$, $\chi^2 = 0.02$, $p = 0.88$, $\varphi = -0.01$), opiates ($df = 1$, $\chi^2 = 2.01$, $p = 0.16$, $\varphi = 0.09$), and PCP ($df = 1$, $\chi^2 = 2.01$, $p = 0.16$, $\varphi = 0.08$). Insufficient data exist to analyze LSD individually.

- Examined in χ^2, the difference in frequencies between arrest-related sudden deaths for people with a history of chronic drug abuse compared to deaths not involving a history of chronic drug abuse is insufficiently large to establish statistical significance ($df = 1$, $\chi^2 = 0.81$, $p = 0.37$, $\varphi = -0.03$). The difference in history of chronic drug abuse is also insufficiently large to establish statistical significance in logit models one and two ($z = 0.55$ and $z = 0.47$).

- When examined in isolation by χ^2, the difference in frequencies between arrest-related sudden deaths for people exhibiting excited delirium compared to people without excited delirium is sufficiently large to establish statistical significance ($df = 1$, $\chi^2 = 16.79$, $p < 0.01$, $\varphi = 0.24$). The logit models also calculate statistically significant differences ($z = 3.01$ and $z = 3.37$). Arrest-related deaths occur more frequently following application of a TASER ECD than in non-ECD cases.

- When examined in isolation by χ^2, the difference in frequencies between arrest-related sudden deaths for people with alcohol in their systems compared to people without alcohol is insufficiently large to establish statistical significance ($df = 1$, $\chi^2 = 0.02$, $p = 0.89$, $\varphi = 0.01$). Both logit models also calculate statistically insignificant differences ($z = 0.26$ and $z = 0.17$).

- When examined in isolation by χ^2, the difference in frequencies between arrest-related sudden deaths for people with a history of chronic alcohol abuse compared to people without a history of chronic alcohol abuse is sufficiently large to establish statistical significance ($df = 1$, $\chi^2 = 9.61$, $p < 0.01$, $\varphi = 0.18$), meaning ECD-proximate deaths are less likely than non-ECD deaths to involve people with a history of alcohol abuse. The logit models also calculate statistically significant differences ($z = -2.43$ and $z = -2.37$).

- When examined in isolation by χ^2, the difference in frequencies between arrest-related sudden deaths for people with mental illness compared to people without a mental illness is sufficiently large to establish statistical significance ($df = 1$, $\chi^2 = 13.78$, $p < 0.01$, $\varphi = 0.21$), meaning ECD-proximate deaths are more likely than non-ECD deaths to involve people with mental illness. Logit model one also calculates a statistically significant difference ($z = 2.81$). However, the mental illness and psychotropic medications variables are collinear (adjusted LR $\chi^2(1) =. 100.24$). Combining the two variables into one variable for logit model two, the difference becomes insufficiently large to establish statistical significance ($z = -1.43$).

- When examined in isolation by χ^2, the difference in frequencies between arrest-related sudden deaths for people taking psychotropic medications compared to people without psychotropic medications is insufficiently large to establish statistical significance ($df = 1$, $\chi^2 = 0.24$, $p = 0.63$, $\varphi = 0.03$). Logit model one also calculates a statistically insignificant difference ($z = -1.86$).

- In the csQCA truth table, 24 case configurations emerge from the 32 causal configurations possible for five dichotomous variables.

- The csQCA truth table cannot be resolved of conflicting configurations, so prime implicants cannot be deduced.

- Of the eight significant configurations with frequency cell counts of ten or more, all are conflicted.

- Only three of the eight significant configurations are more likely to be involved in an ECD-proximate death than they are to be involved in a non-ECD death. One of those configurations contains no condition pertinent to high-risk group theory. The other two configurations contain ExDS in combination with drugs or with drugs and cardiovascular disease.

- Cardiovascular disease and drugs do not appear in any configuration more likely to be involved in an ECD-proximate death, except for configurations that interact with ExDS.

Table 20, Summary of Significance Findings, lists the probabilities or the z-scores for each statistical calculation. An asterisk notes statistically significant findings.

Table 20. Summary of Findings

	χ^2 Model	Logit Models	
		Model 1	Model 2
	$p =$	$z =$	$z =$
AGE	* 0.03	-1.33	-1.43
SEX	*<0.01	1.77	1.75
RACE	0.78	-0.17	0.18
CVD	0.35	-0.11	0.11
ICD	-	0.73	-
DAP	0.15	-1.92	*-2.06
HDA	0.37	0.55	0.47
ExDS	*<0.01	* 3.01	* 3.37
ETOH	0.89	0.26	0.17
HCAA	*<0.01	*-2.43	*-2.37
MT	*<0.01	* 2.81	-
PMED	0.63	-1.86	-
MNTL	-	-	1.43
AP	0.88	-	-
CP	0.11	-	-
MP	0.88	-	-
OP	0.11	-	-
PP	0.16	-	-

* denotes significant at $\alpha \leq 0.05$, $|z| \geq 1.96$

CHAPTER 6

Implications and Conclusions

Arrest-related sudden deaths are rare events, occurring approximately 1.54 times per 100,000 arrests. An arrest-related sudden death is a death that occurs following a collapse within 24 hours after an initial arrest or detention. The death must be unexpected, must not be the result of trauma or injury that a layperson could readily discern needs medical attention, and must follow a sudden change in clinical condition or the beginning of symptoms from which the deceased does not recover. This study examines a sample of 300 cases from the 1,060 such deaths in the United States over the period January 1, 2006 through December 31, 2011.

On average, arrest-related sudden deaths decreased 15.26 deaths per year from 2006 through 2011. Non-ECD deaths decreased 11.89 deaths per year, and ECD-proximate deaths decreased 3.37 deaths per year. The ratio of non-ECD deaths to ECD-proximate deaths ranged from a high of slightly more than 2:1 in 2007 to a low of 1:1 in 2008. The cause of the decrease is not clear from the data in this study. What is evident, however, is that although deaths in both groups are decreasing non-ECD deaths are decreasing more rapidly than ECD-proximate deaths.

ECD-proximate deaths constituted 39.4 percent of all arrest-related sudden deaths. In the six law enforcement agencies with the most arrest-related sudden deaths, ECD-proximate deaths constituted 27.0 percent of those cases. In previous studies on use-of-force, officers employed a TASER ECD in between 22 percent (Smith, Kaminski, Alpert, Fridell, MacDonald, and Kubu, 2009) and 48.8 percent (Gau, et al., 2010) of all use-of-force events. Consequently, the percentage of deaths following the application of an ECD falls within the range of their employment in use of force applications. If the ECD posed a significant risk of death, one would anticipate that the rate of death would be greater than the rate of use of that force option. This does not appear to be the case, but one must take care not to interpret these percentages too liberally. The physiological attributes of sudden arrest-related deaths is likely to be quite different from the physiological attributes in non-fatal use-of-force events. However, the proportion of the involvement of TASER ECDs in arrest-related sudden deaths appears to be roughly equivalent to the proportion of their involvement in all use-of-force events. The range is wide, so additional research on use of all force options needs to be conducted to obtain more accurate data.

High-risk group theory postulates that elderly people, young children, people with pre-existing cardiovascular disease, people with pacemakers and ICDs, people under the influence of drugs (amphetamines, cocaine, LSD, marijuana, opiates, and/or PCP) or with a history of drug abuse, people intoxicated from alcohol or with a history of chronic alcohol abuse, people under extreme psychological distress or who exhibit signs of excited delirium, people who are mentally ill or taking psychotropic medications, people subjected to repeated or multiple applications, and pregnant women are at a heightened risk of serious injury or death following the application of a TASER ECD. Multiple applications and pregnancy are not examined in this study, but there is no evidence to support the other tenets of the theory in this sample, with the possible exception of ExDS.

AGE

In previous studies of arrest-related deaths, the mean age of all arrest-related deaths of 35.7 years is about the same as the mean age in studies of ECD-proximate deaths, which is between 34.8 and 35.9 years. In the current study, the mean age of all arrest-related sudden deaths is 37.8 years, or about 2.1 years older than the previous studies. Part of that difference could be that previous arrest-related death studies include police shootings and suicides, which are not included in this study. The difference could be a product of differences in age of arrest-related sudden deaths and officer-involved shootings or suicides, or it could be a product of sample error.

The mean age of ECD-proximate deaths in this study is 36.8 years, or 0.9 to 2.4 years older than previous studies. The mean age of the

300-case sample is even older (37.2 years). The reason for this difference is not determinable from available data, but the difference between the population and the sample is not sufficiently large to conclude that the difference is anything more than sample error. Insufficient data published in the previous studies prevent a determination of whether the differences between previous studies and the current study are statistically significant.

Examined as a variable independently from the other predictive variable, ECD–proximate deaths are 1.5 years younger than non-ECD deaths in the population and 2.67 years younger than non-ECD deaths in the sample, those differences being statistically significant. However, in both logit models, when controlling for other predictive variables, the difference in ages between the groups is insufficiently large to establish statistical significance.

The range of ages between ECD-proximate deaths and non-ECD deaths is also similar. Ages for non-ECD deaths range from 17 years of age to 85 years of age (68 years). Ages for ECD-proximate deaths range from 16 years of age to 87 years of age (71 years). Kroll, et al., (2009) calculated that ECDs pose no significant risk for people who weigh more than 29.3 pounds, or approximately the 50th percentile weight of a 28.5-month-old male child (National Center for Health Statistics, 2013). Arguments of appropriateness aside, the use of a TASER ECD without deleterious effect is documented on a child as young as eight years old (Hult, 2013) and on an adult as old as 94 (*Associated Press*, 2008). Consequently, evidence from previous studies and from the data in this study do not support the high-risk group theory of additional risk of death for the very young or the very old.

SEX

Males constitute the clear majority of arrest-related deaths. In previously published studies, males are between 93.3 percent and 96.3 percent of arrest-related deaths. In the current study, males are 94.2 percent of all arrest-related deaths in the population and 93.7 percent in the sample. For ECD-proximate deaths, males are between 95.8 percent and 97.4 percent in previous studies. In the current study, males are 98.1 percent of the population and 97.3 percent of the sample.

Why men constitute such a huge majority of ECD-proximate deaths is not discernible from the data in this study. An unlikely hypothesis is that an ECD affects males differently than females. A more likely explanation is that officers feel compelled to use more aggressive tactics, such as the use of ECDs, on men who are physically more capable of resisting arrest or detention than are women. That hypothesis is speculative, but it warrants additional research. It is well-established in the medical literature that men die younger and more frequently than women from almost all causes.

Examined by χ^2 independently from the other predictive variables, sex data from the sample indicates that ECD-proximate deaths more frequently involve males than females. The difference is statistically significant, but the effect size is small. In the logit models, however, while controlling for other predictive variables, the difference in sex in the sample is insufficiently large to establish statistical significance.

RACE

Although it is not a tenet of high-risk group theory, the effects of race and ethnicity are often examined in criminological and medical literature. A brief analysis of race/ethnicity is appropriate in this study because of its potential interaction on the other variables of high-risk group theory. Whites comprise 41.6 percent of the non-ECD deaths, more than any other race or ethnicity. Blacks, however, have the most ECD-proximate deaths with 46.0 percent. When examined by χ^2 analysis using four categorical designations for race, the difference between non-ECD deaths and ECD-proximate deaths is not sufficiently large to conclude that the difference is more than sample error. When designated as a dichotomous variable of White = 0 and all other races/ethnicities = 1 for the logit models, the difference in race remains statistically insignificant in both models. It is clear from the data in this sample that race/ethnicity does not contribute to greater risk of death from the application of a TASER ECD.

CARDIOVASCULAR DISEASE

The second most frequently occurring variable of high-risk group theory in the sample is the presence of cardiovascular disease. The mean age of the 164 cases from the sample (54.7 percent) with cardiovascular disease was 41.0 years, which is 2.75 years older than the mean age of the sample. Analyzed through χ^2 and in both logit models, the difference in non-ECD and ECD-proximate cases is statistically insignificant for people with cardiovascular diseases. When viewed through the significant configurations in csQCA, cardiovascular disease is associated more frequently with non-ECD deaths than with ECD-proximate deaths. Only when cardiovascular disease interacts with ExDS does it become more frequent in ECD-proximate deaths, but that association appears to be due more to the influence of ExDS than of cardiovascular disease.

Of the human model experiments with TASER ECDs, none demonstrates a cardiovascular effect. Moreover, metabolic studies on humans demonstrate that the use of an ECD is less likely than other force options to induce catecholamine release or metabolic acidosis resulting in adverse cardiac effects. Considering the findings of those TASER effect studies with the findings in this study, it appears that the use of an ECD on people with cardiovascular disease is less risky than other force options. However, this study does not examine the effects of force options other than an ECD. Law enforcement officers commonly use more than one force option when subduing a resting subject. More research on the interaction of other force options and cardiovascular disease is necessary to establish the relative risks.

PACEMAKERS AND ICDS

Autopsy reports document only two cases in the sample with ICDs, one of which was a non-ECD death and the other was an ECD-proximate death. Insufficient data from this sample exist for analysis of the variable.

DRUGS

The presence of drugs is the most frequently occurring variable in the study. Toxicology reports demonstrate that 73.0 percent of cases in the study have drugs in their systems at autopsy. More non-ECD cases (115) than ECD-proximate cases (104) present with drugs. When examined independently as a single variable through χ^2, which includes all six drugs examined in this study, the difference in frequencies between arrest-related sudden deaths involving drugs following application of TASER ECDs compared to deaths not involving an ECD is insufficiently large to establish statistical significance. That relationship holds true for individual analyses of amphetamine, cocaine, marijuana, opiates, and PCP. Insufficient data exist to analyze LSD individually.

In logit model one, the difference in non-ECD and ECD-proximate deaths involving drugs is insufficiently large to conclude that the difference is more than sampling error. In logit model two, which dropped the ICD variable and combined the mental illness and psychotropic variables into one variable, the presence of drugs became a statistically significant factor, although the differences in z-scores is very small (-1.92 and -2.06). Logit models one and two indicate that it is less risky to use a TASER ECD than to use other force options on a person intoxicated with drugs (O.R. 0.54 and 0.53, respectively).

It appears that cocaine is the drug primarily responsible for the statistical significance of drugs in logit model two. Previous studies on the effect of a TASER ECD on cocaine-intoxicated animals demonstrate that cocaine provides protection from the stimulation of ectopic heartbeats. Considering those animal model studies with the results of this study, it appears that the use of an ECD on a cocaine-intoxicated person is less risky than other force options. However, this study does not examine the effects of force options other than an ECD. Law enforcement officers commonly use more than one force option when subduing a resting subject. More research on the interaction of other force options and intoxication on cocaine or other drugs is necessary to establish the relative risks.

When viewed through the significant configurations in csQCA, drugs are associated more frequently with non-ECD deaths than with ECD-proximate deaths. Only when drugs interact with ExDS and cardiovascular disease does the condition become more frequent in ECD-proximate deaths, but that association is more likely due to the influence of ExDS than of drugs.

In 35 cases, the medical examiner or coroner notes that the deceased has a history of drug abuse. In 32 cases, those observations are concurrent with drugs in the body. Examined through χ^2 and through logit models one and two, the difference in non-ECD and ECD-proximate deaths is not sufficiently large to conclude that the difference is any more than sample error.

EXCITED DELIRIUM

Excited delirium is not a specific disease or derangement directly observable during autopsy. Instead, ExDS is a constellation of conditions manifesting as a combination of delirium, psychomotor agitation, anxiety, hallucinations, speech disturbances, disorientation, violent and bizarre behavior, insensitivity to pain, elevated body temperature, and extraordinary strength.

Medical examiners and coroners identified ExDS in 77 arrest-related sudden deaths, of which 23 are non-ECD cases, and 54 are ECD-proximate deaths. Viewing that variable singularly through χ^2, the difference is sufficiently large to conclude that it is statistically significant. Additionally, both logit models calculate a statistically significant difference. *Viewed through csQCA, only three significant configurations are more likely to appear in ECD-proximate deaths than in non-ECD deaths. One of those three configurations contains no variable of high-risk group theory. The other two contain ExDS and drugs, and none of the significant configurations that are more likely to appear in non-ECD deaths contains ExDS. Arrest-related deaths involving drug-induced ExDS occur more frequently following application of a TASER ECD than they occur in non-ECD cases.* Cases of ExDS induced by mental illness do not appear in the significant case configurations of the csQCA truth table.

This finding does not necessarily mean that an ECD is more likely to cause a death in an ExDS event, as one cannot make a causal statement based only on retrospective data. Possibly, whatever physiological attributes generate an ExDS event render that person more susceptible to sudden death when exposed to an ECD. An alternative explanation is that people who experience symptoms of ExDS are more physical and more difficult to subdue, so officers are far more likely to use more aggressive tactics, such as the use of an ECD, to subdue them.

Another possible explanation arises from the way medical examiners or coroners report autopsy results. In reading the reports, it becomes apparent that there are two philosophies of what to include in the report. Some pathologists take information provided by law enforcement investigators, family members, and witnesses and include that information in the body of the autopsy. These reports are information-based reports. Other pathologists include only what they observe of the body at the time of autopsy and what they see on medical records supplied from other medical institutions, such as the deceased's doctor or a hospital. There reports are observation-based reports. Because ExDS is not observable at autopsy, observation-based reports will include no mention of the conditions or features described above, and, consequently, no diagnosis of ExDS. Simultaneously, unless evidence in the form of wires or barbs from a TASER ECD cartridge accompany the body, observation-based reports will not mention the use of an ECD. Thus, information-based reports are more likely to associate the use of an ECD with ExDS than are observation-based reports. This reporting difference could account for the difference in observations of ExDS between non-ECD death and ECD-proximate death groups. Regardless of the cause, the significant findings on ExDS raise many critical questions ripe for additional research.

ALCOHOL

The presence of alcohol appears to have no effect on the outcome of the use of a TASER ECD as predicted by the limited literature. Examined through χ^2 analysis and both logit models, the differences between non-ECD and ECD-proximate deaths is insufficiently large to conclude that the differences are more than sampling error. Viewed through csQCA, alcohol does not appear in any of the substantial configurations that appear more frequently in ECD-proximate deaths, although it does appear in the one configuration that occurs with equal frequency in both groups.

One interesting result was the finding regarding a history of chronic abuse of alcohol. Of the 22 cases wherein the medical examiner or coroner recorded a history, 18 of them were non-ECD deaths. When viewed through χ^2 analysis and through both logit models, the difference between non-ECD and ECD-proximate deaths involving people with a history of chronic alcohol abuse is sufficiently large to conclude that it is not a product of sampling error. A history of chronic alcohol abuse does not appear in any of the significant configurations in csQCA.

The reason for this significant finding is not clear from the data. However, the logit model calculations indicate that deaths occur less frequently following use of a TASER ECD on people with a history of chronic alcohol abuse than in deaths in non-ECD cases (O.R. 0.23 and 0.24). Some physical effects of chronic alcohol abuse, such as cirrhosis of the liver, are observable at autopsy. If, however, chronic alcohol abuse is not manifested as an observable anatomical malady, there is no post-mortem test for it. That presents a special issue in analyzing that variable. Unless there is documentation of a previous diagnosis of chronic alcohol abuse, or a family member or close friend can inform the pathologist that the deceased has a history of alcohol abuse, the pathologist cannot diagnose the condition. This finding raises interesting questions that warrant further research.

MENTAL ILLNESS

In 29 cases, medical examiners or coroners report that the deceased is mentally ill or has a history of mental illness. Of those cases, toxicology reports indicate that 13 are taking medications for the illness, seven have drugs in their systems, and three have alcohol in their systems. Eleven are diagnosed with ExDS. When mental illness is examined singularly through χ^2, the difference between non-ECD and ECD-proximate deaths is sufficiently large to conclude that it is statistically significant. In logit model one, where mental illness is examined as a single variable, the difference between non-ECD and ECD-proximate deaths, while controlling for the other predictive variables, is sufficiently large to conclude that the difference is more than sampling error. However, in logit model two, where mental illness is combined with psychotropic medications to form a single variable, the difference is not sufficiently large to conclude that the difference is more than sampling error.

Mental illness is not observable at autopsy, and that presents a special issue in analyzing that variable. Unless there is documentation of a previous diagnosis of mental illness, or a family member or close friend can inform the pathologist that the deceased has a history of mental illness, the pathologist cannot diagnose the illness, as there is no post-mortem test for mental illness. That could explain why toxicology tests showed the presence of psychotropic medications in five of the deceased, but the medical examiner or coroner does not diagnose mental illness. It might be that an ECD affects the mentally ill differently than it affects other people, or it might be that the mentally ill cannot judge when to abandon their resistance, and, consequently, more aggressive tactics, such as the use of an ECD, are necessary to subdue them. Regardless, the conflicting findings raise critical questions that warrant further research.

AGREEMENT BETWEEN ANALYTICAL METHODS

The three analytical methods used to test the research hypotheses, testing individual variables through t-test or χ^2 analysis, testing multiple variables through logistic regression, or case configuration analysis through csQCA, produced strongly consistent results. Although the statistically significant results in individual tests of age and sex disappeared in the logit models that controlled for other predictive variables, that is a common result when comparing individual testing and regression analysis. Variables with differences that proved to be statistically insignificant also failed to appear as causal conditions that occurred more frequently in ECD-proximate deaths than in non-ECD deaths when viewed through csQCA. These results lead to one apparent conclusion—non-ECD deaths and ECD-proximate deaths are similar in physiological attributes, and there is little, if any, evidence to support the belief that people exposed to a shock from a TASER ECD are at greater risk of death because of age, sex, race, previous cardiovascular disease, drugs, alcohol, or mental illness. Evidence that ExDS occurs more frequently following the use of an ECD is not conclusive, but it certainly warrants additional research.

POLICY IMPLICATIONS OF THE RESULTS

The medical literature is rife with studies demonstrating that people with cardiovascular disease, people suffering mental illness, and people intoxicated on drugs or on alcohol are at greater risk of sudden death. Therefore, it is reasonable to expect these attributes to appear in arrest-related sudden death cases regardless of whether a TASER ECD was involved. Unknown is whether the use of TASER ECDs and other weapons or tactics exacerbate or mitigate these risks. Nonetheless, many agencies are establishing policies that restrict the use of ECDs during such high-risk group encounters.

In Great Britain, the Association of Chief Police Officers (2005) published guidelines that advised officers, whenever possible, to discuss use of force options with a mental health professional before using a TASER ECD on a person who exhibits violent behavior, or who suffers from a mental disorder or illness. They also suggested that when it is apparent a subject has an existing medical condition or is under the influence of drugs, that police officers assess those risk factors before determining the appropriate force option.

The International Association of Chiefs of Police (2010) published a model TASER ECD policy that refers to high-risk groups as *sensitive population groups*. Included in the model policy's definition of sensitive population groups are children, the elderly, the medically infirm, pregnant women, and users of a cardiac pacemaker. Although the model policy does not prohibit the use of a TASER ECD on someone in a sensitive population group, it suggests that officers restrict the use of an ECD on such persons to those exceptional circumstances where the potential benefit reasonably outweighs the risks and concerns.

The Police Executive Research Forum (PERF), a non-profit police research organization, was the first national organization to publish a set of recommended guidelines for the use of ECDs (Cronin and Ederheimer, 2006). Although they did not specifically articulate high-risk group theory in their set of 52 guidelines, PERF advised that officers generally should not use ECDs against pregnant women, elderly persons, young children, or visibly frail persons unless exigent circumstances existed. They also urged officers to be aware of the higher risk of sudden death for people under the influence of drugs and for people who exhibit symptoms associated with excited delirium, but they did not connect that increased risk specifically to the use of TASER ECDs.

Five years later, acting jointly with the United States Department of Justice, PERF revised the guidelines, increasing to 53 the recommendations (Police Executive Research Forum and U.S. Department of Justice, 2011). PERF recommended training personnel to use ECDs for one standard cycle and then evaluate the situation to determine whether additional cycles are necessary. They also recommended that training protocols should emphasize multiple applications or continuous cycling of an ECD resulting in an exposure longer than 15 seconds, whether continuous or cumulative, could increase the risk of serious injury or death. PERF reiterated its suggestion that officers should not use ECDs against pregnant women, elderly persons, young children, and visibly frail persons, and they again urged that officers be aware that there is a higher risk of sudden death for subjects under the influence of drugs and for subjects exhibiting symptoms associated with excited delirium.

Thomas, Collins, and Lovrich (2011) analyzed 124 municipal police agency policies that existed in 2009 comparing them for compliance with the PERF guidelines. They determined that 63 percent of the policies prohibited using ECDs on pregnant women, 45 percent prohibited use on the elderly, 50 percent prohibited use on children, and 60 percent prohibited use on other individuals in high-risk groups.

Policies that restrict the use of TASER ECDs compel officers to consider other options to subdue a resisting subject. The officers must forgo the use of the ECD in favor of other less-lethal options, such as pepper spray, batons, and physical force, or immediately escalate to the use of lethal force, such as firearms. Also, because officers cannot easily determine high-risk group vulnerabilities in a person they do not know and have never before met, they must approach all encounters as though the suspects are members of a high-risk group, which severely limits the officers' tactical options.

The potential for fatal adverse effects on high-risk groups when using other less-lethal tactics and methods versus the potential for fatal adverse effects on high-risk groups following the use of a TASER ECD is currently unknown. Therefore, it is also unknown whether more restrictive policies regarding the use of TASER ECDs will result in increased or decreased mortality in high-risk groups. Restrictive policies based upon the uncorroborated theory of high-risk groups could result in law enforcement agencies and officers ultimately bearing greater liability for claims of wrongful death or excessive use of force.

Many law enforcement agencies have begun to re-examine their policies on the use of ECDs on people in high-risk groups, but there is little evidence to suggest that restricting the use of ECDs on will have any significant effect on reducing arrest-related sudden deaths. Based on the results of this study, restricting the use of TASER ECDs on people with pre-existing cardiovascular disease, on people intoxicated on drugs, on people who are intoxicated on alcohol, or on people with mental illness will have little effect in reducing arrest-related sudden deaths. Conversely, *the data indicate that use of an ECD reduces the risk of arrest-related sudden deaths for people intoxicated on cocaine or who have a history of chronic alcohol abuse.* The current literature indicates that use of ECDs reduces injuries to officers and suspects.

Consequently, **restrictions will likely increase non-fatal injuries to officers and suspects without the concomitant benefit of reducing deaths**. Permissive policies regarding use of an ECD are likely to decrease arrest-related deaths for people intoxicated with drugs or who have a history of alcohol while simultaneously reducing injuries to officers and suspects.

The results related to ExDS, however, indicate an increased risk of death following application of an ECD. Further research is necessary to clarify why, but, in the meantime, officers should consider using other force options, whenever possible, on subjects who display symptoms of ExDS. Restricting the use of the ECD in cases of ExDS might reduce ECD-proximate deaths, but that effect is not certain. Whether any reduction in deaths is due to officers using the ECD less frequently will have to be determined with further research.

LEGAL IMPLICATIONS OF THE RESULTS

Despite the several arrest-related sudden deaths that have followed the application of TASER ECDs, several federal circuit courts of appeals have ruled that their use does not constitute deadly force. The 6th Circuit Court of Appeals has ruled that a TASER ECD is a non-lethal weapon (*United States v. Fore*, 2007). The 7th Circuit has recognized "the important role that non-lethal, hands-off means—including [TASER] guns—play in maintaining discipline and order within detention facilities (*Lewis v. Downey*, 2009:476)." The 8th Circuit has ruled that the use of a TASER ECD "is more than a non-serious or trivial use of force but less than deadly force (*McKenney v. Harrison*, 2011:362). The 9th Circuit has stated, "We are not convinced that the use of an X26 involves deadly force (*Marquez v. City of Phoenix*, 2012:1176)." The 11th Circuit has also ruled that a TASER ECD "is a non-deadly weapon commonly carried by law enforcement (*Fils v. City of Aventura*, 2011:1276, n. 2)."

In the United States, "Fourth Amendment jurisprudence has long recognized that the right to make an arrest or investigatory stop necessarily carries with it the right to use some degree of physical coercion or threat thereof to effect it (*Graham v. Connor*, 1989:396)." The Supreme Court has ruled "*all* (emphasis in the original) claims that law enforcement officers have used excessive force—deadly or not—in the course of an arrest, investigatory stop, or other 'seizure' of a free citizen should be analyzed under the Fourth Amendment and its 'reasonableness' standard (*Graham v. Connor*, 1989:365)." The courts must examine the totality of circumstances at the time of the arrest or detention to determine whether an officer used any greater force than was reasonably necessary under the circumstances (*Graham v. Connor*, 1989; *Tennessee v. Garner*, 1985; *Saucier v. Katz*, 2001). "The 'reasonableness' of a particular use of force must be judged from the perspective of a reasonable officer on the scene, rather than with the 20/20 vision of hindsight (*Graham v. Connor*, 1989:396)."

"The 'reasonableness' inquiry in an excessive force case is an objective one: the question is whether the officers' actions are 'objectively reasonable' in light of the facts and circumstances confronting them, without regard to their underlying intent or motivation (*Graham v. Connor*, 1989:397)." However, "[t]he test of reasonableness under the Fourth Amendment is not capable of precise definition or mechanical application (*Bell v. Wolfish*, 1979:559)." The Supreme Court has rejected attempts "to craft an easy-to-apply legal test in the Fourth Amendment context," and it has, instead, acknowledged, "[I]n the end we must still slosh our way through the factbound morass of 'reasonableness' (*Scott v. Harris*, 2007:383)."

The law does not require police officers to calculate the least intrusive means of responding to an exigent situation; it requires only that they act within the range of conduct that the courts identify as reasonable (*Graham v. Connor*, 1989; *Scott v. Henrich*, 1994). Whether officers hypothetically could use less painful, less injurious, or more effective force under a given set of circumstances is not the issue for the court (*Forrester v. City of San Diego*, 1994). However, the law does require officers to consider what other tactics, if any, are available and whether there are clear, reasonable, and less intrusive alternatives to the force employed that could militate against the court finding that the use of force is reasonable (*Bryan v. MacPherson*, 2010).

In *Russo v. City of Cincinnati* (1990), the 6th Circuit Court of Appeals found deployment of a TASER ECD objectively reasonable in incapacitating a potentially homicidal or suicidal individual, even though the individual posed no immediate threat to the officer. Additionally, the single use of an ECD in making the arrest of a suspect who appeared hostile, belligerent, and uncooperative, and who repeatedly refused to comply with a police officer's commands did not amount to excessive force (*Draper v. Reynolds*, 2004).

There is no case law holding that the use of ECDs is *per se* unconstitutional (Kedir, 2007). However, the courts have offered guidance on the limits of what they will consider as reasonable force in circumstances invoking aspects of high-risk group theory. "[W]here it is or should be apparent to the officers that the individual involved is emotionally disturbed, that is a factor that must be considered in determining, under *Graham*, the reasonableness of the force employed (*Deorle v. Rutherford*, 2001:1283)." A person's "emotionally disturbed status may be relevant to the trial court's determination of objective reasonableness (*Ludwig v. Anderson*, 1995:472)." In *Ludwig*, the 8th Circuit Court of Appeals, in part, justified its decision based on the training manual for the law enforcement agency involved.

The courts have forewarned that the physical or psychological condition of an individual affects what the court considers to be reasonable use of force. In *Cruz v. City of Laramie* (2001), the 10th Circuit Court of Appeals found that the use of hog tie restraints on an individual with diminished capacity was a violation of the Fourth Amendment because it was an unreasonable use of force given the situation. The Court explained that diminished capacity can be the result of severe intoxication, drug abuse, a discernible mental illness, or any other condition apparent to the officers at the time that would make the application of a hog-tie restraint likely to result in significant risk to the individual's health or well-being. In *Gregory v. County of Maui* (2008) the 9th Circuit Court of Appeals adopted the 10th Circuit Court's conclusion that the status of someone suffering from a mental illness is relevant to the determination of what is an objectively reasonable use of force.

These rulings have potentially serious consequences regarding liability under 42 U.S.C § 1983 and associated state statutes for officers who use TASER ECDs on high-risk group individuals and for the governmental entities that employ them. The federal appellate courts have already accepted that several conditions suspected in high-risk group theory indicate diminished capacity, including intoxication, drug abuse, and mental illness. A viable argument can also be made that preexisting cardiovascular disease and signs of ExDS constitute "any other condition apparent" that would make the use of a TASER ECD likely to result in "significant risk to the individual's health or well-being."

An example is the decision in the well-publicized case of *Heston, et al. v. City of Salinas, et al.* (2009). Robert Heston, Jr. died after Salinas police officers used a TASER ECD against him. Heston's mother and father and the executor of his estate initiated a civil action against the City of Salinas, against the individual police officers, and against TASER International. The plaintiffs claimed that the police officers violated Heston's civil rights by their use of excessive force. In a product liability claim, the plaintiffs also claimed that TASER International negligently failed to provide warnings that repeated applications of the electrical current in the deployment of an ECD can cause cardiac arrest, especially on persons who are in an agitated or excited physical state. The trial jury returned verdicts in favor of the City of Salinas and the officers, but it returned a verdict against TASER International for negligently failing to warn users of the risks involved in prolonged use. The jury in the case found that, as a consequence of prolonged deployment, Heston suffered acidosis to a degree that caused him to have a cardiac arrest, leading to his death, and it awarded the plaintiffs more than $6,000,000 in damages. The 9th Circuit Court of Appeals later reduced the monetary award on appeal (*Heston, et al. v. TASER International, Inc.*, 2011).

Although the judgment in this case was not against the officers or the city, but rather against the manufacturer, the trial and appellate courts indicated their willingness to accept the multiple applications tenet of high-risk group theory. No doubt, the courts will take notice that high-risk group theory has begun to proliferate in the literature, and they will see that some experts claim the theory to be well-founded, despite the lack of any confirming empirical evidence. Thus, an examination of high-risk group theory is important to adjudicating excessive force and wrongful death claims involving a TASER ECD.

The courts have forewarned what they will consider in deciding the objective reasonableness of a use of force whether an individual is emotionally disturbed (*Deorle v. Rutherford*, 2001; *Ludwig v. Anderson*, 1995), suffering from a mental illness (*Gregory v. County of Maui*, 2008), or suffering from diminished capacity, which can include severe intoxication, drug abuse, a discernible mental illness, or any other condition apparent to the officer that would make that use of force likely to result in significant risk to the individual's health or well-being (*Cruz v. City of Laramie*, 2001). The results reported in this study indicate that the courts should consider that the use of an ECD is no more likely than other force options to result in a significantly increased risk to an individual's health or well-being. In cases of intoxication from drugs, particularly intoxication from cocaine, the use of an ECD is quite possibly less likely to result in a significantly increased risk to an individual's health or well-being. On the other hand, there is an indication that the use of an ECD might result in a significantly increased risk to an individual's health or well-being if that individual is experiencing ExDS, thereby increasing potential liability exposure.

LIMITATIONS OF THE STUDY

The study has limitations worthy of note. First, although extensive research went into constructing the sampling frame, there is no guarantee that all arrest-related sudden deaths were recorded. Indeed, it is highly likely that some cases remained undiscovered. For example, a request for information from the Attorney General's Office in Texas revealed six arrest-related sudden deaths involving the use of a TASER ECD that did not appear in news media databases, on the Internet, or in legal databases. Texas is one of the few states that required reports to the state on all in-custody deaths. It seemed likely that other cases in states without such reporting requirements also escaped publication in news media databases, on the Internet, or in legal databases. Thus, the sampling frame could not be assumed to be the entire population of relevant cases.

Second, 21 states excluded autopsy reports from their respective public information laws. Consequently, cases from which to draw the sample were not missing at random. This limitation adds the potential for bias in the sample.

Third, even though a random sample was extracted from the sampling frame to avoid selection bias, the resulting study population it is not a true random selection. A random selection from a biased population is still biased. Although steps were taken to avoid that possibility, the narrowed field of selection condition could not fully be avoided. Consequently, the question arises of whether the sample in this study is representative of the true population of arrest-related sudden deaths.

Fourth, autopsy reports lacked consistency of form and wording. Different medical examiners and pathologists described similar conditions differently, and they took different approaches to what they included in their reports. Some medical examiners and pathologists recorded only what they observed at autopsy, while some also reported what investigators told them. Consequently, a history of drug abuse, a history of alcohol abuse, or mental illness could have appeared in some reports and not in others. Such differences in the construction of an autopsy report could lead to inconsistent results that coders could not have observed or recorded.

Fifth, not all cardiovascular disease, drug concentrations, or blood alcohol levels created the same physiological threats. For example, for coding purposes a mild coronary occlusion carried the same weight as a cardiovascular disease variable as did a severe myocardial infarct, even though the likelihood of sudden cardiac death associated with each were not equivalent. Creating a ratio scale for such conditions was not realistic in this study considering the knowledge, skills, and experiences of the coders and the researcher, and because of the various ways that medical examiners and pathologists worded their respective reports.

SUGGESTIONS FOR FURTHER RESEARCH

One important avenue for further research concerns the relationship between different force options, such as bodily force, pepper spray, and impact instruments, and their interactions with the physiological attributes of arrest-related sudden death. This study explored only the use of TASER ECDs. Different force options or combinations of options might produce different results. Such research should include an examination of police reports, use of force reports, and autopsy and toxicology records. Additional research is also warranted to explore the interaction of the use of a TASER ECD with ExDS. This research should examine fatal and non-fatal uses of force involving ExDS and the interaction with all force options. This research could be vital to implementing policy and to formulating recommendations on legal decisions regarding the use of force.

CONCLUSIONS

Since the invention of the TASER electronic control device (ECD) in the 1970s, more than 870 people have died worldwide following application of the device. Trying to discover why people died following application of an ECD, researchers have proposed many theories, including direct electro-stimulation of cardiac muscle, interference with breathing, and metabolic derangements resulting in acidosis. Thus far, human experiments have failed to find support for those theories. Recently, a new theory has emerged in the TASER ECD literature that has not been empirically examined—characterized here as the theory of high-risk groups.

High-risk group theory postulates that elderly people, young children, people with pre-existing cardiovascular disease, people with pacemakers and implantable cardioverter-defibrillators, people under the influence of drugs or with a history of drug abuse, people intoxicated from alcohol or with a history of chronic alcohol abuse, people under extreme psychological distress or who exhibit signs of excited delirium, people who are mentally ill or taking psychotropic medications, people subjected to repeated or multiple applications, and pregnant women are at a heightened risk of serious injury or death following application of a TASER ECD. Multiple applications and pregnancy are not tested in this study, although they too are part of the theory of high-risk groups.

What current literature fails to consider is whether physiological characteristics attributable to high-risk group theory might render people more vulnerable to serious injury or death without application of an ECD. This is the first study to examine those differences. For purposes of this study, an arrest-related sudden death is a death that occurs following a collapse within 24 hours after the initial arrest or detention. The death must be unexpected, must not be the result of trauma or injury that a layperson could readily discern requires medical attention, and must follow a sudden change in clinical condition or the beginning of symptoms from which the deceased does not recover. It does not include police shootings and suicides, and it must have occurred in the United States between January 1, 2006 and December 31, 2011.

An experimental or quasi-experimental research design requires applying a shock from a TASER ECD on people who have serious cardiovascular diseases, who are intoxicated on drugs or alcohol, and who are mentally ill. The ethical prohibitions of such a clinical trial are obvious, so this study consists of a retrospective study of autopsy and toxicology reports of 300 arrest-related sudden deaths. Using two very different statistical techniques, inferential statistical techniques (χ^2 and logistic regression analysis) and crisp set Qualitative Comparative Analysis, this study demonstrates no significant difference in the physiological attributes of non-ECD and ECD-proximate groups, except, possibly, for people with a history of chronic alcohol abuse or people who exhibit symptoms of excited delirium syndrome.

A history of chronic alcohol abuse is statically more likely to be associated with non-ECD deaths than with ECD-proximate deaths. The literature offers no guidance in explaining why, but that finding could be an artifact of the different methods used to write autopsy reports. Excited delirium is statically more likely to be associated with ECD-proximate deaths than with non-ECD deaths. However, reasons other than the effect of the ECD might account for that difference. Further research is necessary to determine whether those differences are a product of the effect of a shock from a TASER ECD or the product of research design.

If high-risk group theory were correct, one would expect to see the requisite physiological attributes associated more often with ECD-proximate deaths than with non-ECD deaths. However, there is no evidence in this sample that cardiovascular disease, intoxication from drugs, a history of drug abuse, intoxication from alcohol, a history of chronic alcohol abuse, mental illness, or psychotropic medications are more often associated with ECD-proximate deaths than with non-ECD arrest-related sudden deaths.

Search Terms

Arrest-related death	Arrest-related, died
Batons death	Batons died
Booking desk, death	Booking desk, died
Canine died	Canine death
Chemical spray, death	Chemical spray, died
Custody death	Death in custody
Death while in custody	Death while in police custody
Died in police custody	Died while in police custody
Died while in custody	Died after police
Evaded arrest, death	Evaded arrest, died
Excessive force, death	Excessive force, died
Holding cell, death	Holding cell, died
Inmate death	Inmate died
K-9, died	K-9, death
OC spray, died	OC spray, death
Pepper spray, died	Pepper spray, death
Police brutality, died	Police brutality, death
Resisted arrest, died	Resisted arrest, death
TASER death	TASER died
Stun gun, death	Stun gun, died
Unresponsive police died	Unresponsive police death
Use of force, death	Use of force, died
Wrongful death, police	Wrongful death, deputy

APPENDIX B
Coding Instrument

Demographic Factors

Reference #	Age	Sex
Race/Ethnicity	Height	Weight

TASER ECD

Cardiovascular Disease

Pacemakers or Implantable Cardioverter-Defibrillators

Drugs of Abuse Present

Amphetamines	Cocaine	LSD
Marijuana	Opiates	PCP

History of Drug Abuse

Amphetamines	Cocaine	LSD
Marijuana	Opiates	PCP

Excited Delirium

Alcohol Present

History of Chronic Alcohol Abuse

Mentally Ill

[ ]

Psychotropic Medications

[ ]

Respiration

[ ]

Metabolic Disorders

[ ]

Notes, Concerns, and Questions

[ ]

APPENDIX C

Coding Instrument Instructions

Thank you for agreeing to assist with my research by coding autopsy reports. Attached are coding instruments for each of 300 autopsy reports. Following are instructions on how to complete the instruments. Please remember that accuracy in coding is more important than speed, and there should an appropriate code in every box on the instrument.

DEMOGRAPHIC FACTORS

Reference # – You will receive a worksheet with the names corresponding to all of the autopsy reports. Next to each name on that worksheet is a number ranging from 001 to 300 that corresponds with the name. List the reference number on the coding instrument by writing all three numbers. For example, you would list reference number 6 as 006 and reference number 32 as 032. Do not put the person's name on the coding instrument.

Age – The age for the person is the age the coroner or medical examiner lists on the autopsy report. List the age in whole numbers only. Do not add fractions or decimal places to the age.

Sex – All autopsy reports should list the deceased as either male or female. Indicate male by the capital letter M. Indicate female by the capital letter F.

Race/Ethnicity – The coroner or medical examiner should list a race and/or ethnicity on every report. Indicate Asian or Oriental by the capital letter A. Indicate Black or African/American by the capital letter B. Indicate Hispanic by the capital letter H. Indicate White or Caucasian by the capital letter W. Indicate any other race or ethnicity by the capital letter O.

163

Height – Indicate height in inches by writing the whole number only. Do not add fractions or decimal places to the height. Do not add abbreviations for inches.

Weight – Indicate weight in pounds by writing the whole number only. Do not add fractions or decimal places to the weight. Do not add abbreviations for pounds.

TASER ECD

If the autopsy report mentions the use of a TASER brand name ECD, indicate by using the numeric character 1. If there is no reference to the use of a TASER ECD, indicate by using the numeric character 0. If there is a reference to a stun gun, electroshock device, or neuromuscular incapacitation device, but no reference to the brand name TASER, indicate by using the numeric character 0, but include a comment in the notes section.

CARDIOVASCULAR DISEASE

If the autopsy report indicates any of the following conditions in the diagnosis, as the cause of death, or as a contributing factor to the death, indicate by using the numeric character 1:

- Aortic stenosis
- Atherosclerosis
- Atrial fibrillation
- Atrial flutter
- Atrial myxoma
- Atrioventricular block
- Congestive heart failure
- Coronary artery disease
- Dilated cardiomyopathy
- Hypertrophic cardiomyopathy
- Hypoplasia
- Ischemic heart disease
- Long QT syndrome
- Mitral stenosis
- Mitral valve prolapse
- Multifocal atrial tachycardia
- Myocardial infarction
- Myocarditis
- Premature atrial contractions
- Restrictive cardiomyopathy
- Septal defects
- Sinus bradyarrhythmia
- Sinus tachycardia
- Supraventricular tachycardia
- Tricuspid regurgitation
- Tricuspid stenosis
- Wolff-Parkinson-White syndrome.

If the autopsy report does not mention any of the above conditions, indicate with the numeric character 0.

COMMONLY ABUSED RECREATIONAL DRUGS PRESENT

Amphetamines – If the autopsy report refers to the presence of amphetamine, methamphetamine, methylenedioxyamphetamine, or methylenedioxymethamphetamine, indicate with the numeric character 1. If the autopsy report does not mention any of the above compounds, indicate with the numeric character 0.

Cocaine – If the autopsy report refers to the presence of cocaine, benzoylecgonine, cocaethylene, or ethylbenzoylecgonine, indicate with the numeric character 1. If the autopsy report does not mention any of the above compounds, indicate with the numeric character 0.

LSD – If the autopsy report refers to the presence of LSD, lysergic acid diethylamide, N-desmethyl-LSD, hydroxy-LSD, 2-oxo-LSD, and 2-oxo-3-hydroxy-LSD, indicate with the numeric character 1. If the autopsy report does not mention any of the above compounds, indicate with the numeric character 0.

Marijuana – If the autopsy report refers to the presence of marijuana, tetrahydrocannabinol, or Δ(delta)-9-tetrahydrocannabinol, indicate with the numeric character 1. If the autopsy report does not mention any of the above compounds, indicate with the numeric character 0.

Opiates – If the autopsy report refers to the presence of heroin, diacetylmorphine, morphine, codeine, 3-monoacetylmorphine, or 6-monoacetylmorphine, indicate with the numeric character 1. If the autopsy report does not mention any of the above compounds, indicate with the numeric character 0.

PCP – If the autopsy report refers to the presence of PCP or phencyclidine, indicate with the numeric character 1. If the autopsy report does not mention any of the above compounds, indicate with the numeric character 0.

HISTORY OF DRUG ABUSE

Amphetamines – If the autopsy report refers to the deceased having a history of amphetamine, methamphetamine, methylenedioxyamphetamine, or methylenedioxymethamphetamine abuse, indicate with the numeric character 1. If the autopsy report does not mention any history of abuse involving the above compounds, indicate with the numeric character 0.

Cocaine – If the autopsy report refers to the deceased having a history of cocaine abuse, indicate with the numeric character 1. If the autopsy report does not mention any history of cocaine abuse, indicate with the numeric character 0.

LSD – If the autopsy report refers to the deceased having a history of LSD abuse, indicate with the numeric character 1. If the autopsy report does not mention any history of LSD abuse, indicate with the numeric character 0.

Marijuana – If the autopsy report refers to the deceased having a history of marijuana abuse, indicate with the numeric character 1. If the autopsy report does not mention any history of marijuana abuse, indicate with the numeric character 0.

Opiates – If the autopsy report refers to the deceased having a history of heroin, codeine or morphine abuse, indicate with the numeric character 1. If the autopsy report does not mention any history of opiate abuse, indicate with the numeric character 0.

PCP – If the autopsy report refers to the deceased having a history of PCP abuse, indicate with the numeric character 1. If the autopsy report does not mention any history of PCP abuse, indicate with the numeric character 0.

EXCITED DELIRIUM

If the autopsy report indicates any of the following mental illnesses or disorders in the diagnosis, as the cause of death, or as a contributing factor to the death, indicate by using the numeric character 1:

- Agitated delirium
- Cocaine induced delirium
- Drug induced delirium
- Excited delirium

If the autopsy report does not mention any of the above conditions, indicate with the numeric character 0.

ALCOHOL PRESENT

If the autopsy report indicates the presence of alcohol or ethanol in any amount in the deceased, indicate by using the numeric character 1. If the autopsy report does not mention alcohol, indicate with the numeric character 0.

HISTORY OF CHRONIC ALCOHOL ABUSE

If the autopsy report indicates a history of chronic alcohol abuse, indicate by using the numeric character 1. If the autopsy report does not mention a history of alcohol abuse, indicate with the numeric character 0.

MENTAL ILLNESSES

If the autopsy report indicates any of the following mental illnesses or disorders in the diagnosis, as the cause of death, or as a contributing factor to the death, indicate by using the numeric character 1:

- Schizophrenia
- Bipolar disorder
- Depression.

If the autopsy report does not mention any of the above conditions, indicate with the numeric character 0.

PSYCHOTROPIC MEDICATIONS

If the autopsy report indicates the presence of any of the following medications, indicate by using the numeric character 1:

- Aripiprazole
- Chlorpromazine
- Clozapine
- Fluoxetine
- Olanzapine
- Fluphenazine
- Haloperidol
- Loperidone
- Loxapine
- Molindone
- Paliperidone
- Perphenazine
- Pimozide
- Quetiapine
- Risperidone
- Thioridazine
- Thiothixene
- Trifluoperazine
- Ziprasidone

If the autopsy report does not mention any of the above medications, indicate with the numeric character 0.

RESPIRATION

If the autopsy report indicates any of the following conditions in the diagnosis, as the cause of death, or as a contributing factor to the death, indicate by using the numeric character 1:

- Anoxia
- Asphyxia
- Hypercapnia
- Hypoxemia
- Hypoxia.

If the autopsy report does not mention any of the above conditions, indicate with the numeric character 0.

METABOLIC DISORDERS

If the autopsy report indicates any of the following conditions in the diagnosis, as the cause of death, or as a contributing factor to the death, indicate by using the numeric character 1:

- Acidosis
- Alkalosis
- Hypercalcemia
- Hyperkalemia
- Hypernatremia
- Hyperthermia
- Hypocalcemia
- Hypokalemia
- Hyponatremia
- Ketoacidosis.

If the autopsy report does not mention any of the above conditions, indicate with the numeric character 0.

NOTES, CONCERNS, AND QUESTIONS

If you have questions or concerns regarding any autopsy report, there is a box on the coding instrument in which to record them. Please do not discuss your observations with the other coders.

Again, thank you for volunteering to assist with my research.

STATA Regression Model Tables

LOGIT MODEL ONE

. logit ecd age sex race cvd icd dap hda exds etoh hcaa mt pmed
Iteration 0:   log likelihood = -207.24933
Iteration 1:   log likelihood = -183.04132
Iteration 2:   log likelihood = -182.63326
Iteration 3:   log likelihood = -182.63228
Iteration 4:   log likelihood = -182.63228

Logistic regression

		Number of obs	=	299
		LR chi^2(12)	=	49.23
		Prob > chi^2	=	0.00
Log likelihood = -182.63228		Pseudo R^2	=	0.1188

ECD	Coef.	Std. Err.	z	P>|z|
AGE	-.017376	.013054	-1.33	0.183
SEX	1.159966	.655239	1.77	0.077
RACE	-.044607	.263697	-0.17	0.866
CVD	-.030135	.268430	-0.11	0.911
ICD	1.164287	1.585940	0.73	0.463
DAP	-.620646	.323722	-1.92	0.055
HDA	.230284	.419297	0.55	0.583
EXDS	.941944	.312667	3.01	0.003
ETOH	.081344	.316793	0.26	0.797
HCAA	-1.468250	.605112	-2.43	0.015
MT	2.268083	.807406	2.81	0.005
PMED	-1.605405	.864542	-1.86	0.063
_CONS	-.200705	.883731	-0.23	0.820

. logistic ecd age sex race cvd icd dap hda exds etoh hcaa mt pmed

Logistic regression		Number of obs	=	299
		LR chi^2(12)	=	49.23
		Prob > chi^2	=	0.0000
Log likelihood = -182.63228		Pseudo R^2	=	0.1188

ECD	Odds Ratio	Std. Err.	z	P>|z|
AGE	.982774	.0128294	-1.33	0.183
SEX	3.189826	2.090098	1.77	0.077
RACE	.956373	.252193	-0.17	0.866
CVD	.970315	.260462	-0.11	0.911
ICD	3.203637	5.080776	0.73	0.463
DAP	.537597	.174032	-1.92	0.055
HDA	1.258958	.527878	0.55	0.583
EXDS	2.564962	.801980	3.01	0.003
ETOH	1.084744	.343639	0.26	0.797
HCAA	.230328	.139375	-2.43	0.015
MT	9.660863	7.800242	2.81	0.005
PMED	.200808	.173607	-1.86	0.063

LOGIT MODEL TWO

. logit ecd age sex race cvd dap hda exds etoh hcaa mntl
Iteration 0: log likelihood = -207.24933
Iteration 1: log likelihood = -187.87400
Iteration 2: log likelihood = -187.81334
Iteration 3: log likelihood = -187.81326
Iteration 4: log likelihood = -187.81326

Logistic regression		Number of obs	=	299
		LR chi2(10)	=	38.87
		Prob > chi^2	=	0.0000
Log likelihood = -187.81326		Pseudo R^2	=	0.0938

ECD	Coef.	Std. Err.	z	P>|z|
AGE	-.017474	.012205	-1.43	0.152
SEX	1.030767	.623482	1.65	0.098
RACE	.045271	.258362	0.18	0.861
CVD	.028902	.262352	0.11	0.912
DAP	-.641533	.312119	-2.06	0.040
HDA	.191475	.409460	0.47	0.640
EXDS	1.034792	.307136	3.37	0.001
ETOH	.052349	.312477	0.17	0.867
HCAA	-1.414783	.597726	-2.37	0.018
MNTL	.624046	.436061	1.43	0.152
_CONS	-.136970	.843480	-0.16	0.871

. logistic ecd age sex race cvd dap hda exds etoh hcaa mntl

Logistic regression			Number of obs	=	299
			LR chi^2(10)	=	38.87
			Prob > chi^2	=	0.0000
Log likelihood = -187.81326			Pseudo R^2	=	0.0938

ECD		Odds Ratio	Std. Err.	z	P>$|z|$
AGE	|	.982678	.011993	-1.43	0.152
SEX	|	2.803215	1.747755	1.65	0.098
RACE	|	1.046312	.270327	0.18	0.861
CVD	|	1.029323	.270045	0.11	0.912
DAP	|	.526485	.164326	-2.06	0.040
HDA	|	1.211035	.495870	0.47	0.640
EXDS	|	2.814522	.864439	3.37	0.001
ETOH	|	1.053743	.329270	0.17	0.867
HCAA	|	.242978	.145235	-2.37	0.018
MNTL	|	1.866464	.813892	1.43	0.152

Glossary

Acidosis – An abnormal increase in blood acidity.

Adrenal glands – An endocrine gland located above each kidney that secretes epinephrine and steroids.

Adrenocorticotropic hormone – A hormone of the anterior pituitary that stimulates the production of steroids in the cortex of the adrenal glands.

Afferent sensory neurons – Nerves that carry impulses from receptors or sense organs towards the central nervous system.

Alkalosis – A pathologic condition due to accumulation of base in, or loss of acid from, the body.

Alpha-amylase – A salivary enzyme that hydrolyzes starch.

Anisotropy – The tendency of electric current to follow the grain of skeletal muscle.

Anode – The positive electrode or pole to which negative ions are attracted.

Anoxia – A condition characterized by an absence of oxygen supply to an organ or a tissue.

Anticholinergic – A substance that blocks the neurotransmitter acetylcholine in the central and the peripheral nervous system.

Arrhythmia – A problem with the rate or rhythm of the heartbeat, which can beat too fast, too slow, or with an irregular rhythm.

Arrhythmogenic – Capable of inducing arrhythmias.

Asphyxia – A condition in which an extreme decrease in the amount of oxygen in the body accompanied by an increase of carbon dioxide leads to loss of consciousness or death.

Asthma – A chronic inflammatory disease of the airways.

Asystole – The absence of contractions of the heart.

Atrial fibrillation – An irregularity in heartbeat arrhythmia caused by involuntary contractions of small areas of heart-wall muscle.

Axisymmetric – Having symmetry around an axis.

A-ά motor neurons – Nerve fibers responsible for inducing muscle contractions.

A-δ neural fibers – Nerve endings responsible for temperature and pain sensations.

Benzoylecgonine – A metabolite of cocaine.

β-blocker – A class of drugs that target beta-receptors and weaken the effects of stress hormones.

β-endorphins – A potent endorphin released by the anterior pituitary gland in response to pain, trauma, exercise, or other forms of stress.

Blood oxygen saturation – A relative measure of the amount of oxygen in the blood.

Blood urea nitrogen (BUN)/creatinine ratio – A test to determine kidney function and/or dehydration.

Bradyarrhythmia – A disturbance of the heart's rhythm resulting in a rate less than 60 beats per minute.

Cardiac capture – Beating of the heart in response to external electrical stimuli.

Cardiogenic shock – Inadequate circulation of blood due to primary failure of the ventricles of the heart to function effectively.

Cardiomyopathy – A disease of the heart muscle, usually chronic and with an unknown or obscure cause.

Cardiotoxicity – Drug-induced suppression of heart muscle or its conduction system.

Catecholamine-induced cardiac arrhythmia – Irregular cardiac rhythm caused by naturally occurring compounds in the body such as epinephrine, norepinephrine or dopamine.

Cathode – Negative electrode from which electrons are emitted and to which positive ions are attracted.

Cerebrovascular disease – Any vascular disease affecting cerebral arteries.

Chronaxie – The minimum time required for an electric current double the strength of the rheobase to stimulate a muscle or a neuron.

Clonus – A series of rapid repetitive contractions and relaxations in a muscle during movement.

Computed tomography (CT) – A technique for producing images of cross-sections of the body.

Congestive heart failure – A condition in which the body's tissues are not receiving enough blood and oxygen due to the heart's reduced pumping action.

Coronary ischemia – An inadequate supply of blood and oxygen to meet the metabolic demands of the heart muscle.

Cortisol – A hormone released by the cortex of the adrenal gland when a person is under stress.

Creatine kinase – An enzyme in muscle, brain, and other tissues that catalyzes the transfer of a phosphate group from adenosine triphosphate to creatine, producing adenosine diphosphate and phosphocreatine.

Creatine phosphokinase – An enzyme catalyzing the reversible transfer of phosphate from phosphocreatine to ADP, forming creatine and ATP, which is of importance in muscle contraction.

Diabetes – A chronic syndrome of impaired carbohydrate, protein, and fat metabolism owing to insufficient secretion of insulin or to target tissue insulin resistance.

Diastolic – The phase of blood circulation in which the ventricles are being filled with blood.

Dilatation and curettage – A gynecological procedure in which the cervix is dilated and the lining of the uterus is scraped away.

Dopamine – A neurochemical made in the brain that is involved in many brain activities, including movement and emotion.

Echocardiography – Diagnostic test that uses ultrasound waves to create an image of the heart muscle.

Efferent motor neurons – Nerves that carry impulses away from the central nervous system to effectors such as muscles or glands.

Electrocardiogram – A visual record of the heart's electrical activity.

Electrograms – A record of changes in the electric potentials of specific cardiac loci.

Electroporation – An opening of pores in cellular membranes caused by electrical stimulation.

Endocardium – The thin serous membrane, composed of endothelial and subendothelial tissue, that lines the interior of the heart.

End-tidal carbon dioxide – The level of carbon dioxide in the air exhaled from the body.

End-tidal carbon dioxide – The partial pressure or maximal concentration of carbon dioxide at the end of an exhaled breath.

End-tidal oxygen – The partial pressure or maximal concentration of oxygen at the end of an exhaled breath.

Epicardium – The membrane surrounding the heart.

Epinephrine – A hormone secreted by the adrenal medulla upon stimulation by the central nervous system in response to stress.

Ethybenzoylecgonine – An ethyl ester of cocaine.

Excited delirium syndrome (ExDS) – A condition manifesting as a combination of delirium, psychomotor agitation, anxiety, hallucinations, speech disturbances, disorientation, violent and bizarre behavior, insensitivity to pain, elevated body temperature, and extraordinary strength.

Finite element method – A numerical technique for finding approximate solutions to boundary value problems.

Glucose – A monosaccharide sugar in the blood that serves as the major energy source for the body.

Gout – A form of acute arthritis that causes severe pain and swelling in the joints.

Hematocrit – A measure of how much space in the blood is occupied by red blood cells.

Hypercalcemia – An abnormally high level of calcium in the blood.

Hypercapnia – Excessive carbon dioxide in the blood.

Hypercholesterolemia – High levels of cholesterol.

Hyperkalemia – An abnormally high concentration of potassium ions in the blood.

Hyperkalemia – An excess of potassium in the blood.

Hypernatremia – An excess of sodium in the blood.

Hypertension – High blood pressure.

Hyperthermia – Unusually high body temperature.

Hypertrophy – A growth in size of an organ through an increase in the size, rather than the number, of its cells.

Hyperventilation – Abnormally fast or deep respiration resulting in the loss of carbon dioxide from the blood, thereby causing a decrease in blood pressure.

Hypocalcemia – Abnormally low levels of calcium in blood.

Hypokalemia – Abnormally low potassium levels in the blood.

Hypotension – Low blood pressure.

Hypothalamus-pituitary-adrenal axis – A major part of the neuroendocrine system that controls reactions to stress and regulates many body processes, including digestion, the immune system, mood and emotions, sexuality, and energy storage and expenditure.

Hypothyroidism – Underactive thyroid.

Hypoventilation – Reduced or deficient ventilation of the lungs, resulting in reduced aeration of blood in the lungs and an increased level of carbon dioxide in the blood.

Hypoxemia – Inadequate oxygenation of the blood.

Hypoxia – Insufficient oxygen supply to tissues in the body.

Idioventricular rhythm – A sustained series of impulses propagated by an independent pacemaker within the ventricles with a rate of 20 to 50 beats per minute.

Ketoacidosis – A metabolic state associated with high concentrations of ketone bodies, formed by the breakdown of fatty acids and the deamination of amino acids.

Lactate – A salt or ester of lactic acid.

Lactic acidosis – a physiological condition characterized by low pH in body tissues and blood accompanied by the buildup of lactate.

Maximum heart rate – The fastest rate at which the heart will beat in one minute.

Microvascular disease – Disease of the finer blood vessels in the body, including the capillaries.

Minute ventilation – The total volume of gas in liters exhaled from the lungs per minute.

Mitral valve prolapse – A ballooning of the support structures of the mitral heart valve into the left atrium.

Morphology – The form and structure of an organism considered as a whole.

Myocardial – Pertaining to the muscular tissue of the heart.

Myocardial infarction – The death of a segment of heart muscle caused by a blood clot in the coronary artery interrupting blood supply.

Myocyte – A contractile muscle cell.

Necrosis – Death of cells or tissues through injury or disease.

Norepinephrine – A substance, both a hormone and neurotransmitter, secreted by the adrenal medulla and the nerve endings of the sympathetic nervous system to cause vasoconstriction and increases in heart rate, blood pressure, and the sugar level of the blood.

Partial pressure of carbon dioxide (pCO_2) – The part of total blood gas pressure exerted by carbon dioxide.

Partial pressure of oxygen (pO_2) – The part of total blood gas pressure exerted by oxygen.

Perfusing rhythm – Functioning of the heart muscle sufficient to force blood through the circulatory system.

Peripheral nervous system – That part of the nervous system that lies outside the brain and spinal cord.

pH – A measurement of the acidity or alkalinity of a solution based on the amount of hydrogen ions available.

Phrenic nerve – A nerve that originates in the neck and passes down between the lung and heart to innervate the diaphragm.

Pituitary glands – A small oval gland at the base of the brain in vertebrates that produces hormones that control other glands.

PR interval – The portion of the electrocardiogram between the onset of the P wave (atrial depolarization) and the QRS complex (ventricular depolarization).

Premature ventricular contraction – Contraction of the lower chambers of the heart that occurs earlier than usual because of abnormal electrical activity.

Primary electrical disease – Serious ventricular tachycardia, and sometimes ventricular fibrillation, in the absence of recognizable structural heart disease.

Pseudo-monophasic – A biphasic pulse in which the second phase duration is much greater than the first.

Psychostimulant – An agent that temporarily arouses or accelerates physiological or organic activity.

Pulse oximetry – A non-invasive method allowing the monitoring of the oxygenation of a patient's hemoglobin.

Pulseless electrical activity (PEA) – Continued electrical rhythmicity of the heart in the absence of effective mechanical function.

Purkinje fibers – Any of the specialized cardiac muscle fibers, part of the impulse-conducting network of the heart, that transmit impulses from the atrioventricular node to the ventricles.

QRS duration – The interval from the beginning of the Q wave to the termination of the S wave, representing the time for ventricular depolarization.

QT interval – The time from the beginning of the Q wave to the end of the T-wave, representing the duration of ventricular electrical activity.

QT prolongation – Delayed repolarization of the heart following a heartbeat.

Radiofrequency ablation – Unmodulated, high-frequency, alternating current flow that is applied to heart tissue to raise its temperature and injure cells for the purpose of destroying ectopic foci and accessory pathways.

Resect – Surgically remove a part of a structure or an organ.

Rheobase – The lowest intensity with indefinite pulse duration that stimulates muscles or nerves.

Schizophrenia – Severe psychiatric disorder with symptoms of emotional instability, detachment from reality, and withdrawal into the self.

Serum myoglobin – A test that measures the amount of in the blood.

Sick sinus syndrome – A disorder of the sinus node of the heart, which regulates heartbeat.

Somatic nervous system – That part of the peripheral nervous system that serves the sense organs and muscles of the body wall and limbs and brings about voluntary muscle activity.

Sudden cardiac death – An unexpected and abrupt cessation of cardiac activity.

Sympathetic nervous system – That part of the autonomic nervous system that is active during stress or danger and is involved in regulating pulse and blood pressure, dilating pupils, and changing muscle tone.

Sympathetic-adrenal-medulla axis – Cascade effect of the brain sending signals to the adrenal glands to release stored epinephrine to initiate the fight or flight response.

Sympathomimetic agent – A drug that stimulates the sympathetic nervous system.

Systolic – The phase of blood circulation in which the ventricles are actively pumping blood.

Tachyarrhythmia – A medical condition in which the heartbeat is fast and irregular.

Tachycardia – Abnormally rapid heart rate.

Tidal volume – The volume of gas inhaled and exhaled during one respiratory cycle.

Torsade de pointes (TdP) – Ventricular tachycardia characterized by fluctuation of the QRS complexes around the electrocardiographic baseline.

Trapezius muscle – A large, superficial muscle that spans the neck, shoulders and back.

Troponin I – A contractile protein that increases in serum after myocardial necrosis; a marker of cardiac injury.

Ultrasonography – The use of ultrasound to make images of objects or features that cannot be seen.

Vagal tone – Impulses from the vagus nerve producing inhibition of the heartbeat.

Ventricular fibrillation (VF) – An abnormal and irregular heart rhythm in which there are rapid uncoordinated fluttering contractions of the lower chambers (ventricles) of the heart.

Ventricular tachycardia (VT) – An abnormal heart rhythm that is rapid and regular and that originates from an area of the lower chamber (ventricle) of the heart.

Xiphoid process – The pointed process of cartilage, supported by a core of bone, connected with the lower end of the sternum.

References

Albert, C., Manson, J., Cook, N., Ajani, U., Gaziano, J. & Hennekens, C.
(1999). Moderate alcohol consumption and the risk of sudden cardiac
death among US male physicians. *Circulation, 100*(9):944 – 950.
DOI:10.1161/01.CIR.100.9.944.

Al-Sanouri, I., Dikin, M. & Soubani, A. (2005). Critical care aspects of alcohol
abuse. *Southern Medical Journal, 98*(3): 372 – 381.

Amnesty International. (2004). *Excessive and Lethal Force? Amnesty
International's Concerns about Deaths and Ill-Treatment Involving Police
Use of TASERs.* New York, NY: Author.

Amnesty International. (2006). *Amnesty International's Continuing Concerns
about TASER Use.* New York, NY: Author.

Amnesty International. (2008a). *Less Than Lethal? The Use of Stun Weapons
in US Law Enforcement.* London, England: Author.

Amnesty International. (2008b). *List of Deaths Following Use of Stun Weapons
in US Law Enforcement: June 2001 to 31 August 2008.* London, England:
Author.

Angelidis, M., Basta, A., Walsh, M., Hutson, R. & Strote, J. (2009). Injuries
associated with law enforcement use of conducted electrical weapons.
Academic Emergency Medicine, 16(s1): s229. DOI:10.1111/j.1553-
2712.2009.00391.

Anglen, R. (2004, July 18). TASER safety claim questioned: Medical
examiners connect stun gun to 5 deaths. *The Arizona Republic* (Phoenix,
AZ).

Anglen, R. (2006, January 5). 167 cases of death following stun-gun use. *The
Arizona Republic* (Phoenix, AZ).

Associated Press. (2008, May 2). Police TASER 94-year-old they say killed his
landlord in dispute. Author (Dateline: Oakland, CA).

Association of Chief Police Officers (2005). *Operational Use of TASER Involving Authorized Firearms Officers: Notes for Guidance on Police Use.* London, England: Author.

Azadani, P., Tseng, Z., Ermakov, S., Marcus, G. & Lee, B. (2011). Funding source and author affiliation in TASER research are strongly associated with a conclusion of device safety. *American Heart Journal, 162*(3): 533 – 537. DOI:10.1016/j.ahj.2011.05.025.

Baldwin, D., Nagarakanti, R., Hardy, S., Jain, N., Borne, D., England, A., Nix, E., Daniels, C., Abide, W. & Glancy, D. (2010). Myocardial infarction after TASER exposure. *Journal of the Louisiana State Medical Society, 162*(5): 291 – 295.

Barnes, D., Winslow, J., Alson, R., Johnson, J. & Bozeman, W. (2006). Cardiac effects of the TASER conducted energy weapon. *Annals of Emergency Medicine, 48*(4): s102. DOI:10.1016/j.annemergmed.2006.07.803.

Barnes, D., Winslow, J., Johnson, J., Alson, R., Phillips, C. & Bozeman, W. (2007). Immediate cardiovascular effects of the TASER conducted energy weapon. Winston-Salem, NC: Wake Forest University Baptist Medical Center Faculty Awards Banquet, March 28, 2007.

Barton, A. (2005, August 14). Drugs shadow TASER deaths: 17 of the 27 people who died in Florida after being shocked with a TASER were high on cocaine, officials say. *Palm Beach Post* (West Palm Beach, FL): A1.

Bashian, G., Wagner, G., Wallick, D. & Tchou, P. (2007) Relationship of body mass index (BMI) to minimum distance from skin surface to myocardium: Implications for neuromuscular incapacitating devices (NMID). *Circulation, 116*(16s): 947.

Beason, C., Jauchem, J., Clark, C., Parker, J. & Fines, D. (2009). Pulse variations of a conducted energy weapon (similar to the TASER X26 device): Effects on muscle contraction and threshold for ventricular fibrillation. *Journal of Forensic Sciences, 54*(5): 1113 – 1118.

Bell, L. (1849). On a form of disease resembling some advanced stages of mania and fever, but so contradistinguished from any ordinary observed or described combination of symptoms as to render it probable that it may be overlooked and hitherto unrecorded malady. *American Journal of Insanity, 6*: 97 – 127.

Bernstein, D. (1991, June 12). Inmate claims TASER gun caused miscarriage, sues prison. *Sacramento Bee* (Sacramento, CA): B1.

Bleetman, A., Steyn, R. & Lee, C. (2004). Introduction of the TASER into British policing. Implications for UK emergency departments: An overview of electronic weaponry. *Emergency Medicine Journal, 21*(2): 136 – 140. DOI:10.1136/emj.2003.008581.

Borrego, A. (2011). *Arrest-Related Deaths in the United States: An Assessment of the Current Measurement*. Unpublished master's thesis, Tempe, AZ: Arizona State University.

Bouton, K., Vilke, G., Chan, T., Sloane, C., Levine, S., Neuman, T., Levy, S. & Kolkhorst, F. (2007). Physiological effects of a five second TASER exposure. *Medicine & Science in Sports & Exercise, 39*(5): s323. DOI:10.1249/01.mss.0000274256.70614.ed.

Bozeman, W., Barnes, D., Winslow, J., Johnson, J., Phillips, C. & Alson, R. (2009). Immediate cardiovascular effects of the TASER X26 conducted electrical weapon. *Emergency Medicine Journal, 26*(8): 567 – 570. DOI:10.1136/emj.2008.063560.

Bozeman, W., Teacher, E. & Winslow, J. (2012). Transcardiac conducted electrical weapon (TASER) probe deployments: Incidence and outcomes. *The Journal of Emergency Medicine, 43*(6): 970 – 975. DOI:10.1016/j.jemermed.2012.03.022.

Bozeman, W., Winslow, J. & Hauda, W. (2009). In reply. *Annals of Emergency Medicine, 54*(2): 311 – 312. DOI:10.1016/j.annemergmed.2009.03.015.

Bozeman, W., Winslow, J., Hauda, W., Graham, D., Martin, B. & Heck, J. (2007). Injury profile of TASER electrical conducted energy weapons. *Annals of Emergency Medicine, 50*(3): s65. DOI:10.1016/j.annemergmed.2007.06.356.

Braidwood, T. (2009). *Restoring Public Confidence: Restricting the Use of Conducted Energy Weapons in British Columbia*. Victoria, Canada: Distribution Centre – Victoria.

Bunker, R. (2009). Should police departments develop specific training and policies governing use of multiple TASER shocks against individuals who might be in vulnerable physiological states? *Criminology & Public Policy, 8*(4): 893 – 901. DOI:10.1111/j.1745-9133.2009.00601.

Burch, A. (2011). *Arrest-Related Deaths, 2003 – 2009 Statistical Tables*. Washington, D.C.: Bureau of Justice Statistics.

Burch, A. (2012). Telephone call to the author: May 28, 2012.

Calton, R., Cameron, D., Massé, S. & Nanthakumar, K. (2007). Duration of discharge of neuromuscular incapacitating device and inappropriate implantable cardioverter-defibrillator detections. *Circulation, 115*(20): e472 – 474. DOI:10.1161/CIRCULATIONAHA.107.692129.

Cao, M., Shinbane, J., Gillberg, J., Saxon, L. & Swerdlow, C. (2007). TASER-induced rapid ventricular myocardial capture demonstrated by pacemaker intracardiac electrograms. *Journal of Cardiovascular Electrophysiology,* *18*(8): 876 – 879. DOI:10.1111/j.1540-8167.2007.00881.

Carturan, E., Tester, D., Brost, B., Basso, C., Thiene, G. & Ackerman, M. (2008). Postmortem genetic testing for conventional autopsy-negative sudden unexplained death: An evaluation of different DNA extraction protocols and the feasibility of mutational analysis from archival paraffin-embedded heart tissue. *American Journal of Clinical Pathology, 129*(3): 391 – 397. DOI:10.1309/VLA7TT9EQ05FFVN4.

Chan, T. (2006). Medical overview of sudden in-custody deaths. In Ross, D. & Chan, T. (Eds.). *Sudden Deaths in Custody* (pp. 9 – 14). Totowa, NJ: Humana Press.

Chan, T., Sloane, C., Neuman, T., Levine, S., Castillo, E., Vilke, G., Bouton, K. & Kolkhorst, F. (2007). The impact of the TASER weapon on respiratory and ventilatory function in human subjects. *Academic Emergency Medicine, 14*(s1): s191 – 192. DOI:10.1197/j.aem.2007.03.704.

Chand, M. & Nash, G. (2009). Are TASER guns really safe? *British Journal of Hospital Medicine, 70*(6): 314 – 315. PMID:19516205.

Chugh, S., Kelly, K. & Titus, J. (2000). Sudden cardiac death with apparently normal heart. *Circulation, 102*(6): 649 – 654. DOI:10.1161/01.CIR.102.6.649.

Corruption and Crime Commission. (2010). *The Use of TASER Weapons by Western Australia Police.* Perth, Australia: Author.

Cronin, E. (2013). Sudden cardiac death. In Griffin, B. (Ed.). *Manual of Cardiovascular Medicine, Fourth Edition* (pp. 411 – 423). Lippincott Williams & Wilkins: Philadelphia, PA.

Cronin, J. & Ederheimer, J. (2006). *Conducted Energy Devices: Development of Standards for Consistency and Guidance: The Creation of National CED Policy and Training Guidelines.* Washington, DC: U.S. Department of Justice.

Crumb, W. & Clarkson, C. (1990). Characterization of cocaine-induced block of cardiac sodium channels. *Biophysics Journal, 57*(3): 589 – 599.

Dawes, D. & Kroll, M. (2009). Neuroendocrine effects of CEWs. In Kroll, M. & Ho, J. (Eds.). *TASER Conducted Electrical Weapons: Physiology, Pathology, and Law* (pp. 179 – 185). New York, NY: Springer.

Dawes, D. (2009). Effects of CEWs on respiration. In Kroll, M. & Ho, J. (Eds.). *TASER Conducted Electrical Weapons: Physiology, Pathology, and Law* (pp. 167 – 177). New York, NY: Springer.

Dawes, D., Ho, J. & Miner, J. (2009). The neuroendocrine effects of the TASER X26: A brief report. *Forensic Science International, 183*(1): 14 – 19. DOI:10.1016/j.forsciint.2008.09.015.

Dawes, D., Ho, J., Cole, J., Reardon, R., Lundin, E., Terwey, K., Falvey, D. & Miner, J. (2010). Effect of an electronic control device exposure on a methamphetamine-intoxicated animal model. *Academic Emergency Medicine, 17*(4): 436 – 443. DOI:10.1111/j.1553-2712.2010.00708.

Dawes, D., Ho, J., Johnson, M. & Miner, J. (2007a). 15-second conducted electrical weapon application does not impair basic respiratory parameters, venous blood gases, or blood chemistries and does not increase core body temperature. *Annals of Emergency Medicine, 50*(3): s6. DOI:10.1016/j.annemergmed.2007.06.044.

Dawes, D., Ho, J., Johnson, M. & Miner, J. (2007b). The neuroendocrine effects of the TASER X26 conducted electrical weapon as compared to oleoresin capsicum. *Annals of Emergency Medicine, 50*(3): s132 – 133. DOI:10.1016/j.annemergmed.2007.06.020.

Dawes, D., Ho, J., Johnson, M., Lundin, E., Janchar, T. & Miner, J. (2007). 15-second conducted electrical weapon exposure does not cause core temperature elevation in non-environmentally stressed resting adults. Sorrento, Italy: Fourth Mediterranean Emergency Medicine Congress, September 15 – 18, 2007.

Dawes, D., Ho, J., Johnson, M., Lundin, E., Janchar, T. & Miner, J. (2008). 15-second conducted electrical weapon exposure does not cause core temperature elevation in non-environmentally stressed resting adults. *Forensic Science International, 176*(2): 253 – 257. DOI:10.1016/j.forsciint.2007.09.014.

Dawes, D., Ho, J., Orozco, B., Vogel, E., Nelson, R. & Miner, J. (2010). The respiratory, metabolic, and neuroendocrine effects of a new generation electronic control device. *Academic Emergency Medicine, 17*(s1): s155. DOI:10.1111/j.1553-2712.2010.00743.

Dawes, D., Ho, J., Reardon, R. & Miner, J. (2010). Echocardiographic evaluation of TASER X26 probe deployment into the chests of human volunteers. *American Journal of Emergency Medicine, 28*(1): 49 – 55. DOI:10.1016/j.ajem.2008.09.033.

Dawes, D., Ho, J., Reardon, R., Sweeney, J. & Miner, J. (2010). The physiologic effects of multiple simultaneous electronic control device discharges. *Western Journal of Emergency Medicine, 11*(1): 49 – 56.

Dawson, P. & Moffat, J. (2012). Cardiovascular toxicity of novel psychoactive drugs: Lessons from the past. *Progress in Neuro-Psychopharmacology and Biological Psychiatry, 39*(2): 244 – 252. DOI:10.1016/j.pnpbp.2012.05.003.

Defence Science and Technology Laboratory. (2003). Assessment of the effects of Advanced TASER M26 output on active implantable medical devices. Secretary of State for Defence, London, England. DSTL/PUB20753. In Wilkinson, D. (Ed.) (2006). *Supplement to HOSDB Evaluations of TASER Devices: A Collection of Medical Evidence and Other Source Material*. St. Albans, England: Home Office Police Scientific Development Branch.

Defence Science and Technology Laboratory. (2005). Modelling current flow in the human body from the M26 and X26 TASER devices. Secretary of State for Defence, London, England. DSTL/PUB20755. In Wilkinson, D. (Ed.) (2006). *Supplement to HOSDB Evaluations of TASER Devices: A Collection of Medical Evidence and Other Source Material*. St. Albans, England: Home Office Police Scientific Development Branch.

Defence Scientific Advisory Council Sub-committee on the Medical Implications of Less-Lethal Weapons (DOMILL). (2002). *First DOMILL statement on the medical implications of the use of the M26 Advanced TASER*. London, England: Author.

Defence Scientific Advisory Council Sub-committee on the Medical Implications of Less-Lethal Weapons (DOMILL). (2006). *Second statement on the medical implications of the use of the M26 Advanced TASER*. London, England: Author.

DeMonte, T., Wang, D., Ma, W., Gao, J. & Joy, M. (2009). In-vivo measurement of relationship between applied current amplitude and current density magnitude from 10 mA to 110 mA. *Proceeds from 31st Annual International Conference of the IEEE Engineering in Medicine and Biology Society, 31*(4): 3177 – 3180.

Dennis, A., Valentino, D., Walter, R., Nagy, K., Winners, J., Bokhari, F., Wiley, D., Joseph, K. & Roberts, R. (2007). Acute effects of TASER X26 discharges in a swine model. *Journal of Trauma-Injury Infection & Critical Care, 63*(3): 581 – 590.

Despa, F., Basati, S., Zhang, Z., D'Andrea, J., Reilly, J., Bodnar, E. & Lee, R. (2009). Electromuscular incapacitation results from stimulation of spinal reflexes. *Bioelectromagnetics, 30*(5): 411 – 421. DOI:10.1002/bem.20489.

Di Maio, T. & Di Maio, V. (2006). *Excited Delirium Syndrome: Cause of Death and Prevention*. Boca Raton, FL: CRC Press.

DiFilippo, D. (2012, September 27). Mother sues city after she's TASERed, loses pregnancy. *Philadelphia Daily News* (Philadelphia, PA): 5.

Dyer, A., Stamler, J., Paul, O., Berkson, D., Lepper, M., McKean, H., Shekelle, R., Lindberg, H. & Garside, D. (1977). Alcohol consumption, cardiovascular risk factors, and mortality in two Chicago epidemiologic studies. *Circulation. 56*(6): 1067 – 1074. DOI:10.1161/01.CIR.56.6.1067.

Eastman, A., Metzger, J., Pepe, P., Benitez, F., Decker, J., Rinnert, K., Field, C. & Friese, R. (2008). Conductive electrical devices: A prospective, population-based study of the medical safety of law enforcement use. *Journal of Trauma, Injury, Infection, & Critical Care, 64*(6): 1567 – 1572. DOI:10.1097/TA.0b013e31817113b9.

Eckart, R., Scoville, S., Shry, E., Potter, R. & Tedrow, U. (2006). Causes of sudden death in young female military recruits. *American Journal of Cardiology, 97*(12): 1756 – 1758. DOI:10.1016/j.amjcard.2006.01.036.

Ederheimer, J., Warner, M., Johnson, W. & Fridell, L. (2006). Conducted energy devices: Research on proximate deaths. Los Angeles, CA: American Society of Criminology, November 1 – 4, 2006.

Einarson, A., Bailey, B., Inocencion, G., Ormond, K. & Koren, G. (1997). Accidental electric shock in pregnancy: A prospective cohort study. *American Journal of Obstetrics and Gynecology, 176*(3): 678 – 681.

Eith, C. & Durose, M. (2011). *Contacts between Police and the Public, 2008.* Washington, DC: Bureau of Justice Statistics.

Esquivel, A. & Bir, C. (2008). The development of a model to assess the effects of conducted electrical weapons in a stressful state. *Proceedings of the American Academy of Forensic Sciences, 14*: 270.

Estes, N. (2005). Sudden cardiac arrest from primary electrical diseases: Provoking concealed arrhythmogenic syndromes. *Circulation, 112*(15): 2220 – 2221. DOI: 10.1161/CIRCULATIONAHA.105.573071.

Farnham, F. & Kennedy, H. (1997). Acute excited states and sudden death: Much journalism little evidence. *British Medical Journal, 315*(7116): 1107 – 1108.

Fletcher, G., Flipse, T. & Oken, K. (2004). Exercise and the cardiovascular system. In Fuster, V., Alexander, R. & O'Rourke, R. (Eds.), *Hurst's the Heart, 11th Edition* (pp. 2245 – 2254). New York, NY: The McGraw-Hill Companies.

Fox, A. & Payne-James, J. (2012). Conducted energy devices: Pilot analysis of (non-) attributability of death using a modified Naranjo algorithm. *Forensic Science International, 223*(1 – 3): 261 – 265. DOI:10.1016/j.forsciint.2012.09.016.

Gardner, A., Hauda, W. & Bozeman, W. (2012). Conducted electrical weapon (TASER) use against minors: A shocking analysis. *Pediatric Emergency Care, 28*(9): 873 – 877. DOI:10.1097/PEC.0b013e31826763d1.

Gau, J., Mosher, C. & Pratt, T. (2010). An inquiry into the impact of suspect race on police use of TASERs. *Police Quarterly, 13*(1): 27 – 48. DOI:10.1177/1098611109357332.

Glassman, A. & Bigger, J. (2001). Antipsychotic drugs: Prolonged QTc interval, torsade de pointes, and sudden death. *American Journal of Psychiatry, 158*(11): 1774 – 1782.

Grant, J., Southall, P., Fowler, D., Thomas, E. & Kinlock, T. (2007). Death in custody: A historical analysis. *Journal of Forensic Sciences, 52*(5): 1177 – 1181. DOI: 10.1111/j.1556-4029.2007.00500.x.

Grabetter, F. & Wallnau, L. (2000). *Statistics for the Behavioral Sciences.* Belmont, CA: Wadsworth.

Gunn, J., Evans, M. & Kriger, M. (2009). The systemic role of illicit drugs and their toxicology. In Kroll, M. & Ho, J. (Eds.). *TASER Conducted Electrical Weapons: Physiology, Pathology, and Law* (pp. 327 – 345). New York, NY: Springer.

Haddad, P. & Anderson, I. (2002). Antipsychotic-related QTc prolongation, torsade de pointes and sudden death. *Drugs, 62*(11): 1649 – 1671.

Haegeli, L., Sterns, L., Adam, D. & Leather, R. (2006). Effect of a TASER shot to the chest of a patient with an implantable defibrillator. *Heart Rhythm, 3*(3): 339 – 341. DOI:10.1016/j.hrthm.2005.12.012.

Harris, D. (2010). TASER use by law enforcement: Report of the use of force working group of Allegheny County Pennsylvania. *University of Pittsburgh Law Review, 71*(4): 719 – 763.

Heegaard, W., Halperin, H. & Luceri, R. (2013). Letter by Heegaard et al. regarding article, "Sudden cardiac arrest and death following application of shocks from a TASER electronic control device." *Circulation, 127*(1): e260. DOI:10.1161/CIRCULATIONAHA.112.121988.

Heisig, E. (2011, March 19). Woman claims TASER killed her unborn child. *Houma Today* (Houma, LA). Retrieved March 21, 2011 from http://www.houmatoday.com/article/20110319/ARTICLES/110319423.

Hick, J, Smith, S. & Lynch, M. (1999). Metabolic acidosis in restraint-associated cardiac arrest: A case series. *Academic Emergency Medicine, 6*(3): 239 – 243. DOI:10.1111/j.1553-2712.1999.tb00164.x.

Higginbotham, M., Warnken, B., Snowden, C., Alves, D., Boersma, C., Crawford, C., Hansel, C., Hammack, S., Lopez, C., Johnson, J., McKinney, G., Meekins, K., Pelton, C., Ricks, V. & Warren, M. (2009).

Report of the Maryland Attorney General's Task Force on Electronic Weapons. Baltimore, MD: Office of the Attorney General.

Ho, J. & Dawes, D. (2013). Letter by Ho and Dawes regarding article, "Sudden cardiac arrest and death following application of shocks from a TASER electronic control device." *Circulation, 127*(1): e259. DOI:10.1161/CIRCULATIONAHA.112.118000.

Ho, J. (2005). Sudden in-custody death. *Police, 29*(8): 47 – 48, 50, 54 – 56.

Ho, J. (2009). Can there be truth about TASERs? *Academic Emergency Medicine, 16*(8): 771 – 773. DOI:10.1111/j.1553-2712.2009.00478.

Ho, J., Dawes, D., Bultman, L., Moscati, R., Janchar, T. & Miner J. (2009). Prolonged TASER use on exhausted humans does not worsen markers of acidosis. *American Journal of Emergency Medicine, 27*(4): 413 – 418. DOI:10.1016/j.ajem.2008.03.017.

Ho, J., Dawes, D., Bultman, L., Moscati, R., Skinner, L., Bahr, J., Reardon, R., Johnson, M. & Miner, J. (2007). Physiologic effects of prolonged conducted electrical weapon discharge on acidotic adults. *Academic Emergency Medicine, 14*(s1): s63. DOI:10.1197/j.aem.2007.03.704.

Ho, J., Dawes, D., Bultman, L., Thacker, J., Skinner, L., Bahr, J., Johnson, M. & Miner, J. (2007). Respiratory effect of prolonged electrical weapon application on human volunteers. *Academic Emergency Medicine, 14*(3): 197 – 201. DOI:10.1197/j.aem.2006.11.016.

Ho, J., Dawes, D., Cole, J. & Miner, J. (2008). Human physiologic effects of a civilian conducted electrical weapon application. *Emergency Medicine Australasia, 21*(s1): A28. DOI:10.1111/j.1742-6723.2009.01161.

Ho, J., Dawes, D., Cole, J., Hottinger, J., Overton, K. & Miner, J. (2009). Lactate and pH evaluation in exhausted humans with prolonged TASER X26 exposure or continued exertion. *Forensic Science International, 190*(1): 80 – 86. DOI:10.1016/j.forsciint.2009.05.016.

Ho, J., Dawes, D., Heegaard, W., Calkins, H., Moscati, R. & Miner, J. (2011). Absence of electrocardiographic change after prolonged application of a conducted electrical weapon in physically exhausted adults. *The Journal of Emergency Medicine, 41*(5): 466 – 472. DOI:10.1016/j.jemermed.2009.03.023.

Ho, J., Dawes, D., Johnson, M., Lundin, E. & Miner, J. (2007). Impact of conducted electrical weapons in a mentally ill population: A brief report. *American Journal of Emergency Medicine, 25*(7): 780 – 785. DOI:10.1016/j.ajem.2007.02.030.

Ho, J., Dawes, D., Lapine, A., Bultman, L. & Miner, J. (2008). Prolonged TASER drive stun exposure in humans does not cause worrisome biomarker changes. *Canadian Journal of Emergency Medicine, 10*(3): 274.

Ho, J., Dawes, D., Nelson, R., Lundlin, E., Ryan, F., Overton, K., Zeiders, A. & Miner, J. (2010). Acidosis and catecholamine evaluation following simulated law enforcement "use of force" encounters. *Academic Emergency Medicine, 17*(7): e60 – 68. DOI:10.1111/j.1553-2712.2010.00813.

Ho, J., Dawes, D., Reardon, R., Lapine, A., Dolan, B., Lundin, E. & Miner, J. (2008). Echocardiographic evaluation of a TASER X26 application in the ideal human cardiac axis. *Academic Emergency Medicine, 15*(9): 838 – 844. DOI:10.1111/j.1553-2712.2008.00201.

Ho, J., Dawes, D., Reardon, R., Lapine, A., Olsen, J., Dolan, B. & Miner, J. (2008). Echocardiographic evaluation of human transcutaneous TASER application along the cardiac axis. *Heart Rhythm, 5*(5s): s348. DOI:10.1016/j.hrthm.2008.03.052.

Ho, J., Dawes, D., Reardon, R., Moscati, R., Gardner, R. & Miner, J. (2008). Cardiac and diaphragm ECHO evaluation during TASER device drive stun. Newcastle, Australia: Australasian College for Emergency Medicine Winter Symposium 2008, July 2 – 4, 2008.

Ho, J., Dawes, D., Reardon, R., Strote, S., Kunz, S., Nelson, R., Lundin, E., Orozco, B. & Miner, J. (2011). Human cardiovascular effects of a new generation conducted electrical weapon. *Forensic Science International, 204*(1): 50 – 57. DOI:10.1016/j.forsciint.2010.05.003.

Ho, J., Dawes, D., Ryan, F., Lundin, E., Overton, K., Zeiders, A. & Miner, J. (2009). Catecholamines and troponin in simulated arrest scenarios. Valencia, Spain: The Fifth Mediterranean Emergency Medicine Congress, September 14 – 17, 2009.

Ho, J., Heegaard, W., Dawes, D., Matarajan, S., Reardon, R. & Miner, J. (2009). Unexpected arrest-related deaths in America: 12 months of open source surveillance. *Western Journal of Emergency Medicine, 10*(2): 68 – 73.

Ho, J., Lapine, A., Joing, S., Reardon, R. & Dawes, D. (2008). Confirmation of respiration during trapezial conducted electrical weapon application. *Academic Emergency Medicine, 15*(4): 398. DOI:10.1111/j.1553-2712.2008.00077.

Ho, J., Luceri, R., Lakkireddy, D. & Dawes, D. (2006). Absence of electrocardiographic effects following TASER device application in human volunteers. *Europace, 8*(s1): s22.

Ho, J., Miner, J., Lakkireddy, D., Bultman, L. & Heegaard, W. (2006). Cardiovascular and physiologic effects of conducted electrical weapon discharge in resting adults. *Academic Emergency Medicine, 13*(6): 589 – 595. DOI:10.1197/j.aem.2006.01.017.

Ho, J., Reardon, R., Dawes, D., Johnson, M. & Miner, J. (2007). Ultrasound measurement of cardiac activity during conducted electrical weapon application in exercising adults. *Annals of Emergency Medicine, 50*(3): s108. DOI:10.1016/j.annemergmed.2007.06.406.

Hoffman, L. (2009). ACEP recognizes excited delirium as unique syndrome. *Emergency Medicine News, 31*(11): 4 – 5.

Holden, S., Sheridan, R., Coffey, T., Scaramuzza, R. & Diamantopoulos, P. (2007). Electromagnetic modelling of current flow in the heart from TASER devices and the risk of cardiac dysrhythmias. *Physics in Medicine and Biology, 52*(24): 7193 – 7209.

Hughes, E., Kennett, M., Murray, W., Werner, J. & Jenkins, D. (2007). *Electro-Muscular Disruption (EMD) Bioeffects: A Study of the Effects of Continuous Application of the TASER X26 Waveform on Swine.* An unpublished report from the Institute of Non-Lethal Defense Technologies, The Pennsylvania State University.

Hult, J. (2013, October 9). TASER use on 8-year-old justified, police in S.D. say. *Argus Leader* (Sioux Falls, SD).

Ideker, R. & Dosdall, D. (2007). Can the direct cardiac effects of the electric pulses generated by the TASER X26 cause immediate or delayed sudden cardiac arrest in normal adults? *The American Journal of Forensic Medicine and Pathology, 28*(3): 195 – 201.

Ihejirika, M. (2012, October 5). Suit: Robbins police officers used excessive force, caused miscarriage. *Sun Times* (Chicago, IL). Retrieved October 6, 2012 from http://www.suntimes.com/news/metro/15572117-418/suit-robbins-police-used-excessive-force-caused-misscarriage.html.

International Association of Chiefs of Police. (2006). *Electro-Muscular Disruption Technology: A Nine-Step Strategy for Effective Deployment.* Alexandria, VA: Author.

International Association of Chiefs of Police. (2010). *Electronic Control Weapons Model Policy.* Alexandria, VA: Author.

Isralowitz, R. & Myers, P. (2011). *Illicit Drugs: Health and Medical Issues Today.* Santa Barbara, CA: Greenwood.

Jauchem, J. (2010). Repeated or long-duration TASER electronic control device exposures: Acidemia and lack of respiration. *Forensic Science, Medicine, and Pathology, 6*(1): 46 – 53. DOI:10.1007/s12024-009-9126-4.

Jauchem, J., Beason, C. & Cook, M. (2009). Acute effects of an alternative electronic-control-device waveform in swine. *Forensic Science, Medicine and Pathology, 5*(1): 2 – 10. DOI:10.1007/s12024-009-9076.

Jauchem, J., Cook, M. & Beason, C. (2008). Blood factors of *Sus scrofa* following a series of three TASER electronic control device exposures. *Forensic Science International, 175*(2): 166 – 170. DOI:10.1016/j.forsciint.2007.06.010.

Jauchem, J., Seaman, R. & Klages, C. (2009). Physiological effects of the TASER C2 conducted energy weapon. *Forensic Science, Medicine and Pathology, 5*(3): 189 – 198. DOI:10.1007/s12024-009-9100-1.

Jauchem, J., Sherry, C., Fines, D. & Cook, M. (2006). Acidosis, lactate, electrolytes, muscle enzymes, and other factors in the blood of *Sus scrofa* following repeated TASER exposures. *Forensic Science International, 161*(1): 20 – 30. DOI:10.1016/j.forsciint.2005.10.014.

Karch, S. & Stephens, B. (1999). Drug abusers who die during arrest or in custody. *Journal of the Royal Society of Medicine, 92*(3): 110 – 113. PMID:10396252.

Karch, S. (2006). Cannabis and cardiotoxicity. *Forensic Science, Medicine, and Pathology, 2*(1): 13 – 18. DOI:10.1385/Forensic Sci. Med. Pathol.:2:1:13.

Kargieman, L., Riga, M., Artigas, F. & Celada, P. (2012). Clozapine reverses phencyclidine-induced desynchronization of prefrontal cortex through a 5-HT1A receptor-dependent mechanism. *Neuropsychopharmacology, 37*(3): 723 – 733. DOI:10.1038/npp.2011.249.

Kedir, S. (2006). Stunning trends in shocking crimes: A comprehensive analysis of TASER weapons. *Journal of Law and Health, 20*(2): 357 – 384.

Kershaw, S. (2004, March 7). As shocks replace police bullets, deaths drop but questions arise. *New York Times* (New York, NY): N1, N20.

Khaja, A., Govindarajan, G., McDaniel, W. & Flaker, G. (2008). Effect of stun gun discharges on pacemaker function. *Circulation, 118*(s): 592.

Kim, P. & Franklin, W. (2005). Ventricular fibrillation after stun-gun discharge. *New England Journal of Medicine, 353*(9): 958 – 959.

Koponen, H., Alaräisänen, A., Saari, K., Pelkonen, O., Huikuri, H., Raatikainen, M., Savolainen, M. & Isohanni, M. (2008). Schizophrenia and sudden cardiac death: A review. *Nordic Journal of Psychiatry, 62*(5): 342 – 345. DOI:10.1080/08039480801959323.

Kornblum, R. & Reddy, S. (1991). Effects of the TASER in fatalities involving police confrontation. *Journal of Forensic Sciences, 36*(2): 434 – 448. DOI:10.1520/JFS13046J.

Kraines, S. (1034). Bell's mania. *The American Journal of Psychiatry, 91*(1): 29 – 40.

Kroll, M. (2007). Crafting the perfect shock. *IEEE Spectrum, 12*: 27 – 30.

Kroll, M. (2009). Physiology and pathology of TASER electronic control devices. *Journal of Forensic and Legal Medicine, 16*(4): 173 – 177. DOI:10.1016/j.jflm.2008.12.012.

Kroll, M., Calkins, H., Luceri, R., Graham, M. & Heegaard, W. (2008). Sensitive swine and TASER electronic control devices. *Academic Emergency Medicine, 15*(7): 695 – 696. DOI:10.1111/j.1553-2712.2008.00141.

Kroll, M., Luceri, R. & Calkins, H. (2007). A very interesting case study involving a TASER conducted electrical weapon (CEW) used on a patient with a pacemaker. *Journal of Cardiovascular Electrophysiology, 18*(12): e29 – 30. DOI:10.1111/j.1540-8167.2007.00989.

Kroll, M., Panescu, D., Brewer, J., Lakkireddy, D. & Graham, M. (2009). Weight adjusted meta-analysis of fibrillation risk from TASER conducted electrical weapons. *Proceedings of the American Academy of Forensic Sciences, 15*: 177 – 178.

Kroll, M., Panescu, D., Carver, M., Kroll, R. & Hinz, A. (2009). Cardiac effects of varying pulse charge and polarity of TASER conducted electrical weapons. *Proceeds from 31st Annual International Conference of the IEEE Engineering in Medicine and Biology Society, 31*(4): 3195 – 3198.

Kroll, M., Panescu, D., Hinz, A. & Lakkireddy, D. (2010). A novel mechanism for electrical currents inducing ventricular fibrillation: The three-fold way to fibrillation. Buenos Aires, Argentina: Proceedings from the 32nd Annual International IEEE EMBS Conference, August 31 – September 4, 2010: 1990 – 1996.

Kroll, M., Sweeney, J. & Swerdlow, J. (2006). Theoretical considerations regarding the cardiac safety of law enforcement electronic control devices. *Proceedings of the American Academy of Forensic Sciences, 12*: 139 – 140.

Kukowski, J. (2012). Unpublished e-mail to the author: December 4, 2012.

Kunz, S., Grove, N. & Fischer, F. (2012). Acute pathophysiological influences of conducted electrical weapons in humans: A review of current literature. *Forensic Science International, 221*(1): 1 – 4. DOI:10.1016/j.forsciint.2012.02.014.

Kunz, S., Zinka, B., Fieseler, S., Graw, M. & Peschel, O. (2012). Functioning and effectiveness of electronic control devices such as the TASER M- and

X-series: A review of the current literature. *Journal of Forensic Sciences,*
    57(6): 1591 – 1594. DOI:10.1111/j.1556-4029.2012.02167.
Kupari, M. & Koskinin, P. (1998). Alcohol, cardiac arrhythmias and sudden
    death. In Chadwick, D. & Goode, J. (Eds.). *Alcohol and Cardiovascular*
    Diseases (pp. 68 – 79). New York, NY: John Wiley & Sons, Ltd.
Kutcher, S., Ayer, S., Bowes, M., Ross, J., Sanford, F., Smith, L., Techan, M.
    & Theriault, S. (2009). *Report of the Panel of Mental Health and Medical*
    Experts Review of Excited Delirium. Halifax, Canada: Nova Scotia
    Ministry of Health.
Lakkireddy, D., Biria, M., Baryun, E., Berenbom, L., Pimentei, R., Emert, M.,
    Kreighbaum, K., Kroll, M. & Verma, A. (2008). Can electrical-conductive
    weapons (TASER) alter the functional integrity of pacemakers and
    defibrillators and cause rapid myocardial capture? *Heart Rhythm, 5*(5s):
    s97. DOI:10.1016/j.hrthm.2008.03.042.
Lakkireddy, D., Khasnis, A., Antenacci, J., Ryshcon, K., Chung, M., Wallick,
    D., Kowalewski, W., Patel, D., Micochova, H., Kondur, A., Vacek, J.,
    Martin, D., Natale, A. & Tchou, P. (2007). Do electrical stun guns
    (TASER X26) affect the functional integrity of implantable pacemakers
    and defibrillators? *Europace, 9*(7): 551 – 556.
    DOI:10.1093/europace/eum058.
Lakkireddy, D., Kowalewski, W., Wallick, D., Verma, A., Martin, D.,
    Ryschon, K., Butany, J., Natale, A. & Tchou, P. (2006). Cardiovascular
    safety profile of electrical stun guns (TASER): Impact of point of delivery
    on ventricular fibrillation thresholds, *Heart Rhythm, 3*(5): s249.
Lakkireddy, D., Wallick, D., Ryschon, K., Chung, M., Butany, J., Martin, D.,
    Saliba, W., Kowalewski, W., Natale, A. & Tchou, P. (2006). Effects of
    cocaine intoxication on the threshold for stun gun induction of ventricular
    fibrillation. *Journal of the American College of Cardiology, 48*(4): 805 –
    811. DOI:10.1016/j.jacc.2006.03.055.
Lakkireddy, D., Wallick, D., Verma, A., Ryschon, K., Kowaleski, W., Wazni,
    O., Butany, J., Martin, D. & Tchou, P. (2008). Cardiac effects of electrical
    stun guns: Does position of barbs contact make a difference? *Pacing and*
    Clinical Electrophysiology, 31(4): 398 – 408. DOI:10.1111/j/1540-
    8159.2008.01007.x.
Lange, R. & Hillis, L. (2010). Sudden death in cocaine abusers. *European*
    Heart Journal, 31(3): 271 – 273. DOI:10.1093/eurheartj/ehp503.
Laub, J. (2011). *Study of Deaths Following Electro Muscular Disruption.*
    Washington, DC: Department of Justice.

Lee, B., Vittinghoff, E., Whiteman, D., Park, M., Lau, L. & Tseng, Z. (2009). Relation of TASER (electrical stun gun) deployment to increase in in-custody deaths. *American Journal of Cardiology, 103*(6): 877 – 880. DOI:10.1016/j.amjcard.2008.11.046.

Leitgeb, N., Niedermayr, F., Loos, G. & Neubauer, R. (2011). Cardiac fibrillation risk of TASER X26 dart mode application. *Wiener Mediziniche Wochenschrift, 161*(23 – 24): 571 – 577.

Leitgeb, N., Niedermayr, F., Nuebauer, R. & Loos, G. (2012). Risk of pacemaker patients by TASER X26 contact mode application. *Journal of Electromagnetic Analysis and Applications*, 4(2): 96 – 100. DOI:10.4236/jemaa.2012.42012.

Levine, S., Sloane, C., Chan, T., Dunford, J. & Vilke, G. (2007). Cardiac monitoring of human subjects exposed to the TASER. *Journal of Emergency Medicine, 33*(2): 113 – 117. DOI:10.1016/j.jemermed.2007.02.018.

Levine, S., Sloane, C., Chan, T., Vilke, G. & Dunford, J. (2005). Cardiac monitoring of subjects exposed to the TASER. *Academic Emergency Medicine, 12*(s1): s71. DOI:10.1111/j.1553-2712.2005.tb03828.

Levine, S., Sloane, C., Chan, T., Vilke, G. & Dunford, J. (2006a). Cardiac monitoring of human subjects exposed to the TASER. *Academic Emergency Medicine, 13*(s5): s47. DOI:10.1111/j.1553-2712.2006.tb02227.

Levine, S., Sloane, C., Chan, T., Vilke, G. & Dunford, J. (2006b). Cardiac monitoring of subjects exposed to the TASER. *Prehospital Emergency Care, 10*(1): 130. DOI:10.1080/10903120500444420.

Lindsay, A., Foale, R., Warren, O. & Henry, J. (2005). Cannabis as a precipitant of cardiovascular emergencies. *International Journal of Cardiology, 104*(2): 230 – 232. DOI:10.1016/j.ijcard.2004.10.038.

Link, M. & Estes, N. (2008). Cardiac safety of electrical stun guns: Letting science and reason advance the debate. *Pacing and Clinical Electrophysiology, 31*(4): 395 – 397. DOI:10.1111/j.1540-8159.2008.01007.

Long, J. (1997). *Regression Models for Categorical and Limited Dependent Variables*. Thousand Oaks, CA: Sage Publications.

Lucas, W. & Cairns, J. (2006). Lethality of TASERs – The Canadian experience. American Academy of Forensic Sciences 58th Annual Meeting: Seattle, Washington, February 20 – 25, 2006.

Maddux, S. (2012, December 12). Did TASERing cause LaPorte inmate's miscarriage? *South Bend Tribune* (South Bend, IN).

Maier, A., Nance, P., Price, P., Sherry, C., Reilly, J., Klauenberg, B. & Drummond, J. (2005). *Human Effectiveness and Risk Characterization of the Electromuscular Incapacitation Device—A Limited Analysis of the TASER*. Quantico, VA: The Joint Non-Lethal Weapons Human Effects Center of Excellence.

Mash, D., Duque, L., Pablo, J., Quin, Y., Adi, N., Hearn, W., Hyma, B., Karch, S., Druid, H. & Wetli, C. (2009). Brain biomarkers for identifying excited delirium as a cause of sudden death. *Forensic Science International, 190*(1 – 3): e13 – e19.

McDaniel, W. & Stratbucker, R. (2006). Testing the cardiac rhythm safety of the thoracic application of TASER devices. *Europace, 8*(s1): s23.

McDaniel, W., Stratbucker, R. & Smith, R. (2000). Surface application of the TASER stun guns does not cause ventricular fibrillation in canines. Chicago, IL: *Proceedings of the 22nd Annual International Conference of the IEEE Engineering in Medicine and Biology Society*, July 23 – 28, 2000. Retrieved April 25, 2007 from http://cironline.org/sites/default/files/legacy/files/2000-SurfaceApplicationofTaserStunGunsDoesNotCauseVentricularFibrillation inCanines.pdf.

McDaniel, W., Stratbucker, R., Nerheim, M. & Brewer, J. (2005). Cardiac safety of neuromuscular incapacitating defensive devices. *Pacing and Clinical Electrophysiology, 28*(s1): s284 – 287.

Mehl, L. (1992). Electrical injury from TASERing and miscarriage. *Acta Obstetrica et Gynecologica Scandinavica, 71*(2): 118 – 123.

Meithe, T., Hart, T. & Regoeczi, W. (2008). The conjunctive analysis of case configurations: An exploratory method of discrete multivariate analyses of crime data. *Journal of Quantitative Criminology, 24*(2): 227 – 241.

Mesloh, C., Henych, M., Hougland, S. & Thompson, F. (2005). TASER and less lethal weapons: An exploratory analysis. *Law Enforcement Executive Forum, 5*(5): 67 – 79.

Milroy, C. & Parai, J. (2011). The histopathology of drugs of abuse. *Histopathology, 59*(4): 579 – 593. DOI:10.1111/j.1365-2559.2010.03728.x.

Mirchandani, H., Rorke, L., Sekula-Perlman, A. & Hood, I. (1994). Cocaine-induced agitated delirium, forceful struggle, and minor head injury: A further definition of sudden death during restraint. *American Journal of Forensic Medicine and Pathology, 15*(2): 95 – 99.

Morrison, A. & Sadler, D. (2001). Death of a psychiatric patient during physical restraint. Excited delirium – A case report. *Medicine, Science, and Law, 41*(1): 46 – 50.

Moscati, R., Ho, J., Dawes, D. & Miner, J. (2010). Physiologic effects of prolonged conducted electrical weapon discharge in ethanol-intoxicated adults. *The American Journal of Emergency Medicine, 28*(5): 582 – 587. DOI:10.1016/j.ajem.2009.02.010.

Mumola, C. (2007). *Arrest-Related Deaths in the United States, 2003 – 2005.* Washington, D.C.: Bureau of Justice Statistics.

Munetz, M., Fitzgerald, D. & Woody, M. (2006). Police use of the TASER with people with mental illness in crisis. *Psychiatric Services: A Journal of the American Psychiatric Association, 57*(6): 883. DOI:10.1176/appi.ps.57.6.883.

Murphy, S., Xu, J. & Kochanek, K. (2012). Deaths: Preliminary data for 2010. *National Vital Statistics Reports, 60*(4): 1 – 52.

Nanthakumar, K., Billingsley, I., Massé, S., Dorian, P., Cameron, D., Chauhan, V., Downar, E. & Sevaptsidis, E. (2006). Cardiac electrophysiological consequences of neuromuscular incapacitating device discharges. *Journal of the American College of Cardiology, 48*(4): 798 – 804.

National Center for Health Statistics. (2013). Growth Charts. Atlanta, GA: Centers for Disease Control and Prevention. Retrieved October 14, 2013 from http://www.cdc.gov/growthcharts/html_charts/wtage.htm.

National Institute of Justice. (2008). *Study of Deaths Following Electro Muscular Disruption: Interim Report.* Washington, D.C.: U.S. Department of Justice.

Naunheim, R., Treaster, M. & Aubin, C. (2010). Ventricular fibrillation in a man shot with a TASER. *Emergency Medicine Journal, 27*(8): 645 – 646. DOI:10.1136/emj.2009.088468.

Oakes, A. (2002, June 29). Chula Vista rejects claim of woman shot with TASER: She links stillbirth to actions of police. *Union-Tribune* (San Diego, CA): B2.

O'Brien, A., McKenna, B. & Simpson, A. (2007). Health professionals and the monitoring of TASER use. *Psychiatric Bulletin, 31*(10): 391 – 393. DOI:10.1192/pb.bp.106.014175.

O'Brien, A., McKenna, B., Thom, K., Diesfeld, K. & Simpson, A. (2011). Use of TASERs on people with mental illness: A New Zealand database study. *International Journal of Law and Psychiatry, 34*(1): 39 – 43. DOI:10.1016/j.ijlp.2010.11.006.

Okie S. (2010). A flood of opioids, a rising tide of deaths. *New England Journal of Medicine, 363*(21): 1981 – 1985. DOI:10.1056/NEJMp1011512.

Olmedo, R. (2006). Phencyclidine and ketamine. In Flomenbaum, N., Goldfrank, L., Hoffman, R., Howland, M., Lewin, N. & Nelson, L. (Eds.), *Goldfrank's Toxicologic Emergencies, 8th Edition.* (pp. 1231 – 1243). New York, NY: The McGraw-Hill Companies.

Panescu, D. (2007). Numerical estimation of TASER conducted electrical weapon current flow and effects on human body. Kanazawa, Japan: Bioelectromagnetics Society 29th Annual Meeting, June 10 – 15, 2007.

Panescu, D., Kroll, M. & Stratbucker, R. (2008). Theoretical possibility of ventricular fibrillation during use of TASER neuromuscular incapacitation devices. *Proceeds from 30th Annual International IEEE Engineering in Medicine and Biology Society Conference, 30*(4): 5671 – 5674.

Panescu, D., Kroll, M. & Stratbucker, R. (2009). Medical safety of TASER conducted energy weapon in a hybrid 3-point deployment mode. *Proceeds from 31st Annual International Conference of the IEEE Engineering in Medicine and Biology Society, 31*(4): 3191 – 3194.

Panescu, D., Kroll, M., Efimov, I. & Sweeney, J. (2006). Finite element modeling of electric field effects of TASER devices on nerve and muscle. *Engineering in Medicine and Biology Magazine, IEEE, 1*(1): 1277 – 1279.

Paninski, R., Marshall, M. & Link, M. (2013). ICD oversensing caused by TASER. *Journal of Cardiovascular Electrophysiology, 24*(1): 101. DOI:10.1111/jce.12046.

Park, E., Choi, S., Ahn, J.& Min, Y. (2013). Repetitive TASER X26 discharge resulted in adverse physiologic events with a dose-response relationship related to the duration of discharge in anesthetized swine model. *Journal of Forensic Sciences, 58*(1): 179 – 183. DOI:10.1111/j.1556-4029.2012.02287.

Park, K., Korn, C. & Henderson, S. (2001). Agitated delirium and sudden death: Two case reports. *Prehospital Emergency Care, 5*(2): 214 – 316.

Pasquier, M., Carron, P., Vallotton, L. & Yersin, B. (2011). Electronic control device exposure: A review of morbidity and mortality. *Annals of Emergency Medicine, 58*(2): 178 – 188. DOI:10.1016/j.annemergmed.2011.01.023.

Passiel, T., Halpern, J., Stichtenoth, D., Enrich, H. & Hintzen, A. (2008). The pharmacology of lysergic acid diethylamide: A review. *CNS Neuroscience & Therapeutics 14*(4): 295 – 314. DOI:10.1111/j.1755-5949.2008.00059.x.

Patel, M., Belson, M., Wright, D., Lub, H., Heningere, M. & Miller, M. (2005). Methylenedioxymethamphetamine (ecstasy)-related myocardial hypertrophy: An autopsy study. *Resuscitation, 66*(2): 197 – 202. DOI:10.1016/j.resuscitation.2005.01.020.

Pestaner, J. & Southall, P. (2003). Sudden death during arrest and phencyclidine intoxication. *The American Journal of Forensic Medicine and Pathology, 24*(2): 119 – 122. DOI:10.1097/01.paf.0000064520.90683.5a.

Peters, J. (2006). Sudden death, excited delirium, and issues of force: Part II. *Police and Security News, 22*(3): 1 – 4.

Phillips, M., Robinowitz, M., Higgins, J., Boran, K., Reed, T. & Virmani, R. (1986). Sudden cardiac death in Air Force recruits: A 20-year review. *JAMA: Journal of the American Medical Association, 256*(19): 2696 – 2699.

Pinto, D. & Josephson, M. (2004). Sudden cardiac death. In Fuster, V., Alexander, R. & O'Rourke, R. (Eds.), *Hurst's the Heart, 11th Edition* (pp. 1051 – 1078) New York, NY: The McGraw-Hill Companies.

Pippin, J. (2007). TASER research in pigs not helpful. *Journal of the American College of Cardiology, 49*(7): 731 – 732. DOI:10.1016/j.jacc.2006.11.019.

Police Executive Research Forum & U.S. Department of Justice (2011). *2011 Electronic Control Weapon Guidelines.* Washington, D.C.: Authors.

Pollanen, M., Chiasson, D., Cairns, J. & Young, J. (1998). Unexpected death related to restraint for excited delirium: a retrospective study of deaths in police custody and in the community. *Canadian Medical Association Journal, 158*(12): 1603 – 1607.

Primavesi, R. (2009). A shocking episode: Care of electrical injuries. *Canadian Family Physician, 55*(7): 707 – 709.

Ragin, C. (1987). *The Comparative Method: Moving Beyond Qualitative and Quantitative Strategies.* Berkeley, CA: University of California Press.

Ragin, C. (1999). Qualitative comparative analysis and causal complexity. Health Services Research, 34(5): 1225 – 1239.

Rahko, P. (2008). Evaluation of the skin-to-heart distance in the standing adult by two-dimensional echocardiography. *Journal of the American Society of Echocardiography 21*(6): 761 – 764. DOI:10.1016/j.echo.2007.10.027.

Ranson, D. (2012). Excited delirium: A political diagnosis. *Journal of Law and Medicine, 19*(4): 667 – 672.

Ray, W., Chung, C., Murray, K., Hall, K. & Stein, M. (2009). Atypical antipsychotic drugs and the risk of sudden cardiac death. *The New England Journal of Medicine, 360*(3): 225 – 235. DOI:10.1056/NEJMoa0806994.

Reardon, R. (2009). Echocardiographic effects of the CEW. In Kroll, M. & Ho, J. (Eds.). *TASER Conducted Electrical Weapons: Physiology, Pathology, and Law* (pp. 153 – 161). New York, NY: Springer.

Recinos, R., Miller, B., Hutchinson, M., Llanes, M., Acosta, C., Alayon, A., Armesto, E., Campbell-Dumeus, O., Diblin, T., Edgington, L., Fajardo, L., Geroges, L., Laurenceau, F., Llama, M., Lopez, A., Pruss, O., Ramos, S. Robinette, L., Santos, A. & Thomas, C. (2005). *Final Report of the Miami-Dade Grand Jury: Spring Term A.D. 2005.* In the Circuit Court of the Eleventh Judicial Circuit of Florida in and for the County of Miami-Dade. Retrieved March 2, 2007 from http://www.miamisao.com/publications/grand_jury/2000s/gj2005s.pdf.

Richards, K., Kleuser, L. & Kluger, J. (2008). Fortuitous therapeutic effect of TASER shock for a patient in atrial fibrillation. *Annals of Emergency Medicine, 52*(6): 686 – 688. DOI:10.1016/j.annemergmed.2008.04.023.

Rihoux, B. (2006). Qualitative comparative analysis (QCA) and related systematic comparative methods. *International Sociology, 21*(5): 679 – 706. DOI:10.1177/0268580906067836.

Rihoux, B. & De Meur, G. (2009). Crisp-set qualitative comparative analysis (csQCA). In Rihoux, B. & Ragin, C. (Eds.). *Configurational Comparative Methods: Qualitative Comparative Analysis (QCA) and Related Techniques* (pp. 33 – 68). Thousand Oaks, CA: Sage Publications.

Roberts, J. (2007). Acute agitated delirium from cocaine: A medical emergency. *Emergency Medicine News, 29*(10): 18 – 20.

Robison, D. & Hunt, S. (2005). Sudden in-custody death syndrome. *Topics in Emergency Medicine, 27*(1): 36 – 43.

Ryan, E. (2008). Shocked and stunned: A consideration of the implications of TASERs in Australia. *Current Issues in Criminal Justice, 20*(2): 293 – 302.

Ryan, E. (2011). *Below the Belt: Police Use of Conducted Energy Weapons in Australia.* Unpublished doctoral dissertation, Melbourne, Australia: Monash University.

Sabine, M., Straus, M., Bleumink, G., Dieleman, J., van der Lei, J., Jong, G., Kingma, H., Sturkenboom, M. & Stricker, B. (2004). Antipsychotics and the risk of sudden cardiac death. *Archives of Internal Medicine, 164*(12): 1293 – 1297. DOI:10.1001/archinte.164.12.1293.

Schlosberg, M. (2005). *Stun Gun Fallacy: How the Lack of TASER Regulation Endangers Lives.* San Francisco, CA: American Civil Liberties Union of Northern California.

Sloane, C. & Vilke, G. (2008). Medical aspects of less-lethal weapons. *Law Enforcement Executive Forum, 8*(4): 81 – 94.

Sloane, C., Chan, T., Levine., S., Dunford, J., Neuman, T. & Vilke, G. (2008). Serum troponin I measurement of subjects exposed to the TASER X26. *The Journal of Emergency Medicine, 35*(1): 29 – 32. DOI:10.1016/j.jemermed.2007.08.073.

Sloane, C., Vilke, G., Chan, T., Levine, S. & Dunford, J. (2007). Serum troponin I measurement of subjects exposed to the TASER X26. *Academic Emergency Medicine, 14*(s1): s103 – 104. DOI:10.1197/j.aem.2007.03.704.

Smith, M., Kaminski, R., Alpert, G., Fridell, L., MacDonald, J. & Kubu, B. (2009). *A Multi-Method Evaluation of Police Use of Force Outcomes.* Washington, D.C.: National Institute of Justice.

Smith, P. (2006). An introduction to TASER electronic control devices, history, electricity, electrical stimulation, electrical measurements, and the human body: Expert report of Patrick (Rick) W. Smith in the matter of *Betty Lou Heston, et al. vs. City of Salinas (CA), et al.*, in the United States District Court for the Northern District of California, San Jose Division, Case No. C-05-03658 RS.

Southall, P., Grant, J., Fowler, D. & Scott, S. (2008). Police custody deaths in Maryland, USA: An examination of 45 cases. *Journal of Forensic and Legal Medicine, 15*(4): 227 – 230. DOI:10.1016/j.jflm.2007.10.005.

Standing Advisory Subcommittee on the Use of Force. (2007). *Analysis and Recommendations for a Quebec Police Practice on the Use of Conducted Energy Devices.* Nicolet, Canada: Author.

Starmer, K. & Gordon, J. (2007). *PSNI's Proposed Introduction of TASER: Human Rights Advice.* Belfast, Northern Ireland: Police Service of Northern Ireland.

Stephens, B., Jentzen, J., Karch, S., Wetli, C. & Mash, D. (2004). National association of medical examiners position paper on the certification of cocaine-related deaths. *The American Journal of Forensic Medicine and Pathology, 25*(1): 11 – 13.

Stoughton, C., Pendergrass, T., Zelon, H. & Al-Khatib, A. (2011). *Taking TASERs Seriously: The Need for Better Regulation of Stun Guns in New York.* New York, NY: New York Civil Liberties Union.

Stratbucker, R., Kroll, M., McDaniel, W. & Panescu, D. (2006). Cardiac current density distribution by electrical pulses from TASER devices. *Engineering in Medicine and Biology Magazine, IEEE, 1*(1): 6305 – 6307.

Stratbucker, R., Roeder, R. & Nerheim, M. (2003). Cardiac safety of high voltage TASER X26 waveform. *Proceeds from 25th Annual International Conference of the IEEE Engineering in Medicine and Biology Society, 25*(4): 3261 – 3262.

Stratton, S., Rogers, C., Brickett, K. & Gruzinski, G. (2001). Factors associated with sudden death of individuals requiring restraint for excited delirium. *American Journal of Emergency Medicine, 19*(3): 187 – 191. DOI:10.1053/ajem.2001.22665.

Strote, J. & Hutson, H. (2006). TASER use in restraint-related deaths. *Prehospital Emergency Care, 10*(4): 447 – 450. DOI:10.1080/10903120600884863.

Strote, J. & Hutson, H. (2009). TASER study results do not reflect real-life restraint situations. *American Journal of Emergency Medicine, 27*(6): 747. DOI:10.1016/j.ajem.2009.05.017.

Strote, J., Campbell, R., Pease, J., Hamman, M. & Hutson, R. (2005). The role of TASERs in police restraint-related deaths. *Annals of Emergency Medicine, 46*(3s): 85. DOI:10.1016/j.annemergmed.2005.06.314.

Sun, H. (2007). *Models of VF Probability and Neuromuscular Stimulation after TASER Use in Humans.* Unpublished doctoral dissertation, Madison, WI: University of Wisconsin at Madison.

Sun, H., Haemmerich, S., Rahko, P. & Webster, J. (2010). Estimating the probability that the TASER directly causes human ventricular fibrillation. *Journal of Medical Engineering & Technology, 34*(3): 178 – 191. DOI:10.3109/03091900903509149.

Sun, H., Wu, J., Abdallah, R. & Webster, J. (2005). Electromuscular incapacitating device safety. Prague, Czech Republic: IFMBE Proceedings from the 3rd European Medical and Biological Engineering Conference, November 20 – 25, 2005.

Sweeney, J. (2009). Theoretical comparisons of nerve and muscle activation by neuromuscular incapacitation devices. *Proceeds from 31st Annual International Conference of the IEEE Engineering in Medicine and Biology Society, 31*(4): 3188 – 3190.

Swerdlow, C., Fishbein, M., Chaman, L., Lakkireddy, D. & Tchou, P. (2009). Presenting rhythm in sudden deaths temporally proximate to discharge of TASER conducted electrical weapons. *Academic Emergency Medicine, 16*(8): 726 – 739. DOI:10.1111/j.1553-2712.2009.00432.

Swerdlow, C., Kroll, M., Williams, H., Biria, M., Lakkireddy, D. & Tchou, P. (2008). Presenting rhythm in sudden custodial deaths after use of TASER

electronic control device. *Heart Rhythm, 5*(5s): s44.
DOI:10.1016/j.hrthm.2008.03.041.

Synyshyn, S. (2008). *A Briefing Note on the State of TASERs in Canada: A
Select Review of Medical and Policy Review Literature.* Ottawa, Canada:
The Canadian Association of Police Boards.

Sztajnkrycer, M. & Baez, A. (2005). Cocaine, excited delirium and sudden
unexpected death. *Emergency Medical Services, 34*(4): 77 – 81.

Tchou, P. (2007). Finding the edge of heart safety. *IEEE Spectrum, 12*: 30 – 31.

Tchou, P., Lakkireddy, D. & Wallick, D. (2007). Effects of torso dart position
and cocaine intoxication on TASER induction of ventricular fibrillation.
Proceedings of the American Academy of Forensic Sciences, 13: 423 –
424.

Terrill, W., Paoline, E. & Ingram, J. (2012). *Final Technical Report Draft:
Assessing Police Use of Force Policy and Outcomes.* Unpublished report
submitted to U.S Department of Justice. Retrieved March 6, 2012 from
https://www.ncjrs.gov/pdffiles1/nij/grants/237794.pdf.

Thomas, K., Collins, P. & Lovrich, N. (2011). An analysis of written
conductive energy device policies: Are municipal policing agencies
meeting PERF recommendations? *Criminal Justice Policy Review, 23*(4):
399 – 426. DOI:10.1177/0887403411412372.

Valentino, D., Walter, R., Dennis, A., Margeta, B., Starr, F., Nagy, K., Bokhari,
F., Wiley, D., Joseph, K. & Roberts, R. (2008). TASER X26 discharges in
swine: Ventricular rhythm capture is dependent on discharge vector. *The
Journal of Trauma Injury, Infection, and Critical Care, 65*(6): 1478 –
1487.

Vanga, S., Bommana, S., Phil, M., Kroll., M., Swerdlow, C. & Lakkireddy, D.
(2009). TASER conducted electrical weapons and implanted pacemakers
and defibrillators. *Proceeds from 31st Annual International Conference of
the IEEE Engineering in Medicine and Biology Society, 31*(4): 3199 –
3204.

VanMeenen, K., Cherniack, N., Bergen, M., Gleason, L., Teichman, R. &
Servatius, R. (2010). Cardiovascular evaluation of electronic control
device exposure in law enforcement trainees: A multisite study. *Journal of
Occupational and Environmental Medicine, 52*(2): 197 – 201.
DOI:10.1097/JOM.0b013e3181cc58ba.

VanMeenen, K., Lavietes, M., Cherniack, N., Bergen, M., Teichman, R. &
Servatius, R. (2011). *Respiratory and Cardiovascular Response During
Electronic Control Device (ECD) Exposure in Law Enforcement Trainees.*
Washington, DC: U.S. Department of Justice.

Vearrier, D., Greenberg, M., Miller, S., Okaneku, J. & Haggerty, D. (2012). Methamphetamine: History, pathophysiology, adverse health effects, current trends, and hazards associated with the clandestine manufacture of methamphetamine. *Disease-a-Month, 58*(12): 38 – 89. DOI:10.1016/j.disamonth.2011.09.004.

Vilke, G., Chan, T. & Karch, S. (2013). Letter by Vilke et al. regarding article, "Sudden cardiac arrest and death following application of shocks from a TASER electronic control device." *Circulation, 127*(1): e258. DOI:10.1161/CIRCULATIONAHA.112.119990.

Vilke, G., DeBard, M., Chan, T., Ho, J., Dawes, D., Hall, C., Curtis, M., Costello, M., Mash, D., Coffman, S., McMullen, M., Metzger, J., Roberts, J., Sztajnkrycer, M., Henderson, S., Adler, J., Czarnecki, F., Heck, J. & Bozeman, W. (2011). Excited delirium syndrome (ExDS): Defining based on a review of the literature. *The Journal of Emergency Medicine, 43*(5): 897 – 905. DOI:10.1016/j.jemermed.2011.02.017.

Vilke, G., Johnson, W., Castillo, E., Ederheimer, J., Sloan, C. & Chan, T. (2006). Evaluation of in-custody deaths proximal to use of conductive energy devices. *Annals of Emergency Medicine, 48*(4): s23. DOI:10.1016/j.annemergmed.2006.07.523.

Vilke, G., Sloane, C., Bouton, K., Kolkhorst, F., Levine, S., Neuman, T., Castillo, E. & Chan, T. (2007). Physiological effects of a conducted electrical weapon on human subjects. *Annals of Emergency Medicine, 50*(5): 569 – 575. DOI:10.1016/j.annemergmed.2007.05.004.

Vilke, G., Sloane, C., Levine, S., Neuman, T., Castillo, E. & Chan, T. (2008). Twelve-lead electrocardiogram monitoring of subjects before and after voluntary exposure to the TASER X26. *American Journal of Emergency Medicine, 26*(1): 1 – 4. DOI:10.1016/j.ajem.2007.01.005.

Vilke, G., Sloane, C., Suffecool, A., Kolkhorst, F., Neuman, T., Castillo, E. & Chan, T. (2009). Physiologic effects of the TASER after exercise. *Academic Emergency Medicine, 16*(8): 704 – 710. DOI:10.1111/j.1553-2712.2009.00458.

Vilke, G., Sloane, C., Suffecool, A., Neuman, T., Castillo, E., Kolkhorst, F. & Chan, T. (2007). Physiologic effects of the TASER on human subjects after exercise. *Annals of Emergency Medicine, 50*(3): s55. DOI:10.1016/j.annemergmed.2007.06.325.

Walcott, G. Kroll, M. & Ideker, R. (2011). Ventricular fibrillation threshold of rapid short pulses. Boston, MA: *Proceedings from the 33rd Annual International IEEE EMBS Conference*:255 – 258.

Walter, R., Dennis, A., Valentino, D., Margeta, B., Nagy, K., Bokhari, F., Wiley, D., Joseph, K. & Roberts, R. (2008). TASER X26 discharges in swine produce potentially fatal ventricular arrhythmias. *Academic Emergency Medicine, 15*(1): 66 – 73. DOI:10.1111/j.1553-2712.2007.000012.x.

Wannamethee, G. & Shaper, A. (1992). Alcohol and sudden cardiac death. *British Heart Journal, 68*(5): 443 – 448. DOI:10.1136/hrt.68.11.443.

Webster, J., Will, J., Sun, H., Wu, J., O'Rourke, A., Huebner, S. & Rahko, P. (2006). Can TASERs directly cause ventricular fibrillation? *International Federation for Medical and Biological Engineering Proceedings,* 14: 3307 – 3310.

Wetli, C. & Fishbain, D. (1985). Cocaine-induced psychosis and sudden death in recreational cocaine users. *Journal of Forensic Sciences, 30*(3): 873 – 880. DOI:10.1520/JFS11020J.

Wetli, C., Mash, D. & Karch, S. (1996). Cocaine-associated agitated delirium and the neuroleptic malignant syndrome. *American Journal of Emergency Medicine, 14*(4): 425 – 428.

White, M. & Ready, J. (2007). The TASER as a less lethal force alternative. Findings on use and effectiveness in a large metropolitan police agency. *Police Quarterly, 10*(2): 170 – 191. DOI:10.1177/1098611106288915.

White, M. & Ready, J. (2009). Examining fatal and nonfatal incidents involving the TASER. *Criminology & Public Policy, 8*(4): 865 – 891. DOI:10.1111/j.1745-9133.2009.00600.x.

White, M. & Ready, J. (2010). Police use of the TASER in the United States: Research, controversies, and recommendations. In Knutsson, J. & Kuhns, J. (Eds.), *Police Use of Force: A Global Perspective* (pp. 177 – 187). Santa Barbara, CA: Praeger.

White, M., Ready, J., Riggs, C., Dawes, D., Hinz, A. & Ho, J. (2013). An incident-level profile of TASER device deployments in arrest-related deaths. *Police Quarterly, 16*(1): 85 – 112. DOI:10.1177/1098611112457358.

Whitfield, E. & Lai, A. (2011). *A Force to be Reckoned With: TASER Use and Policies in 20 Arizona Law Enforcement Agencies.* Phoenix, AZ: American Civil Liberties Union of Arizona.

Williams, H. (2008). *TASER Electronic Control Devices and Sudden In-Custody Death: Separating Evidence and Conjecture.* Springfield, IL: Charles C. Thomas, Publisher.

Woodford, N. (2006). Injuries and death resulting from restraint. In Rutty, G. (Ed.). *Essentials of Autopsy Practice: Current Methods and Modern Trends* (pp. 171 – 188). London, England: Springer-Verlag.

World Health Organization. (2010). *International Classification of Diseases.* Geneva, Switzerland: Author. Retrieved October 30, 2011 from http://www.who.int/classifications/icd/en/.

Wu, J., Sun, H., O'Rourke, A., Huebner, S., Rahko, R., Will, J. & Webster, J. (2008). TASER blunt probe dart-to-heart distance causing ventricular fibrillation in pigs. *IEEE Transactions on Biomedical Engineering, 55*(12): 2768 – 2771.

Zipes, D. (2012). Sudden cardiac arrest and death associated with application of shocks from a TASER electronic control device. *Circulation, 125*(20): 2417 – 2422. DOI:10.1161/CIRCULATIONAHA.112.097584.

Cases Cited

Bell v. Wolfish, 441 U.S. 520 (1979).

Bryan v. MacPherson, 630 F.3d 805 (9th Cir. 2010).

Cruz v. City of Laramie, 239 F.3d 1183 (10th Cir. 2001).

Deorle v. Rutherford, 272 F.3d 1272 (9th Cir. 2001).

Draper v. Reynolds, 369 F.3d 1270 (11th Cir. 2004).

Fils v. City of Aventura, 647 F.3d 1272 (11th Cir. 2011).

Forrester v. City of San Diego, 25 F.3d 804 (11th Cir. 1994) (Cert. denied at 513 U.S. 1152).

Globe Newspaper Company v. Chief Medical Examiner, 404 Mass. 132 (1989).

Graham v. Connor, 490 U.S. 386 (1989).

Gregory v. County of Maui, 523 F.3d 1103 (9th Cir. 2008).

Heston, et al. v. TASER International, Inc., et al., 431 Fed. Appx. 586; 2011 U.S. App. LEXIS 9389 (9th Cir. 2011).

Heston, et al. v. City of Salinas, et al., 2009 U.S. Dist. LEXIS 10096, U.S. District Court for the Northern District of California (2009).

Johnstown Tribune Publishing v. Ross, 871 A.2nd 324 (2009).

Lewis v. Downey, 581 F.3d 467 (7th Cir. 2009) (Cert. denied in *Shreffler v. Lewis*, 130 S. Ct. 1936).

Ludwig v. Anderson, 54 F.3d 465 (8th Cir. 1995).

Marquez v. City of Phoenix, 693 F.3d 1167 (9th Cir. 2012).

McKenney v. Harrison, 635 F.3d 354 (8th Cir. 2011).

Russo v. City of Cincinnati, 953 F.2d 1036 (6th Cir. 1992).

Saucier v. Katz, 533 U.S. 194 (2001).

Scott v. Harris, 550 U.S. 372 (2007).

Scott v. Henrich, 39 F.3d 912 (9th Cir. 1994) (Cert. denied at 515 U.S. 1159).

TASER International, Inc. et al. v. Kohler, 2006-11-7421, Summit County, OH, Final Order, (May 2, 2008).

TASER International, Inc. et al. v. Kohler, 2009 Ohio App. LEXIS 1334 (March 31, 2009) (Discretionary appeal not allowed by *TASER International, Inc. v. Kohler*, 2009 Ohio LEXIS 2390 (Ohio, August 26, 2009)).

Tennessee v. Garner, 471 U.S. 1 (1985).

United States v. Fore, 507 F.3d 412 (6th Cir. 2007).

Index

3,4-methylenedioxy-N-
methamphetamine, 27-28
6th Circuit Court of Appeals, 151-
152
7th Circuit Court of Appeals, 151
8th Circuit Court of Appeals, 151-
152
9th Circuit, 151, 153-154
10th Circuit Court of Appeals,
152-153
11th Circuit Court of Appeals, 151
Acidosis, 9, 11, 26, 45, 63, 72, 75-
80, 82-85, 143, 153, 156, 179
Adrenocorticotropic hormone, 75
Afferent sensory neurons, 82
Alcohol, 9-10, 12-13, 16-17, 19,
24-27, 35, 39, 66-67, 81-82,
85, 87, 96, 100-103, 108,
123-125, 128, 131, 133, 135,
140, 146-148, 150, 155-158
Alkalosis, 72
Alpha-amylase, 82-83
American College of Emergency
Physicians, 34
American Medical Association, 33
Amnesty International, 6-8, 12,
183

Amphetamine, 10, 24, 27-28, 66,
95, 115, 117, 131, 134, 140,
143
Methamphetamine, 35
Anisotropy, 40
Arrest-related sudden death, 105,
132
Association of Chief Police
Officers, 148
Asthma, 78
Asystole, 40, 43, 64-65
Atrial fibrillation, 25, 40, 66
Atropine, 65-66
Autonomic hyperarousal state, 35
A-α motor neurons, 3, 51
A-δ neural fibers, 2
Bayer Laboratories, 30
Bell, Luther, 33
Benzoylecgonine.27, 95
Bicarbonate, 73, 76, 78-80
Blood oxygen saturation, 43, 72
Blood urea nitrogen/creatinine
ratio, 78
Boolean algebra, 101
Buprenorphine, 30
Bureau of Justice Statistics, 4, 15,
19, 24, 92
β-blocker therapy, 66
ß-endorphins, 75

Calcium, 77, 178
Calmeil, L. F., 33
Cannabis, 24, 26, 29, 67
Cardiac capture, 28, 46-49, 54-55,
     60, 62-64, 70
Cardiac death, 21-22, 25, 29, 32,
     35, 155
Cardiogenic shock, 28
Cardiomyopathy, 25, 71, 84
Cardiotoxicity, 28
Cardiovascular disease, 5, 11, 13,
     16-17, 19, 21-22, 31, 39, 85,
     87, 97-102, 108, 114, 127-
     128, 133-134, 136, 140, 142-
     144, 148, 150, 153, 155-157
Cardioverter-defibrillator, 12-13,
     17, 19, 67-72, 87, 95, 100,
     102-103, 108, 115-116, 128,
     131, 134, 140, 143
Catecholamine, 35, 76, 84, 143
Causal conditions, 102, 128, 131
Causal configuration, 130, 136
Center for Disease Control, 19
Cerebrovascular disease, 78
Chronaxie, 40-41, 49, 51, 53
CJ-11A, 92
Clonus, 3
Cocaethylene, 27, 95
Cocaine, 7, 10, 24, 26-28, 34-36,
     42, 49, 66, 95-96, 115, 117-
     118, 131, 135, 140, 143-144,
     150, 154
Codeine, 30, 95-96
Computed tomography, 63
Congestive heart failure, 78
Coronary ischemia, 29
Corruption and Crime
     Commission, 13
Cortisol, 82-83

Cover, Jack, 1
Creatine kinase, 78
Creatine phosphokinase, 85
Davidson, G. M., 34
Death in Custody Reporting Act,
     15
Deaths in Custody Reporting
     Program, 4, 19, 23-24, 92
Defence Science and Technology
     Laboratory, 67
Defence Scientific Advisory
     Council Sub-committee on
     the Medical Implications of
     Less-Lethal Weapons, 10-11
Defibrillator, See Cardioverter-
     defibrillator
Department of Defense, 5
Department of Justice, 5-6, 12-13,
     149
Derby, Irving, 34
Diabetes, 78
Diagnostic and Statistical Manual
     of Mental Disorders, 4th
     Edition, 33
Diphenoxylate, 30
Dopamine, 35, 84
Dose-response curves, 50
Drugs, 10-13, 16-17, 19-20, 24-
     25, 30-35, 39, 66, 85, 87, 97,
     100-103, 108, 115-117, 121-
     123, 125, 127-128, 131, 134,
     136, 140, 143-145, 147-150,
     154, 156-157
Echocardiogram, 63
Echocardiograph, 63-64
Echocardiography, 44-48, 55, 60-
     62
Ectopy, 49
Efferent motor neurons, 82

Electrocardiogram, 40, 44-45, 56-
60, 62-63, 66
Electrocardiograms, 44, 46, 57,
58-60, 62, 63
Electrogram, 71
Electro-muscular disruption, 3
Electroporation, 51-54
End tidal oxygen, 74
Endocardium, 41
End-tidal carbon dioxide, 72-74
End-tidal oxygen, 73-74
Epicardium, 40-41, 43, 48
Epinephrine, 35, 42, 44, 65-66, 75,
84
Ethylbenzoylecgonine, 27, 95, 167
Excessive force, 14, 91, 151-154
Excited delirium, 11-12, 14, 17,
19, 33-36, 39, 44, 55, 81, 85,
87, 96-97, 100-103, 108, 122-
123, 125, 127-128, 131, 133,
135-136, 140, 143-150, 153-
154, 156-157
ExDS, See Excited delirium
Federal Bureau of Investigation, 4,
19, 23
Fentanyl, 30
Fourth Amendment, 151, 153
Fundamental law of
electrostimulation, 53
Glucose, 77
Gout, 78
Health Insurance Portability and
Accountability Act, 16, 87
Hematocrit, 75, 77
Heroin, 30, 95-96
Heston, Robert, 153
Hofmann, Albert, 30
Hydrocodone, 30
Hydromorphone, 30

Hypercholesterolemia, 78
Hyperkalemia, 78, 80
Hypertension, 78
Hyperthermia, 26, 35, 75
Hypertrophy, 27-28
Hyperventilation, 72
Hypotension, 45, 76
Hypothalamus-pituitary-adrenal
axis, 75, 82
Hypothermia, 66-67
Hypothyroidism, 78
Hypoventilation, 72
Hypoxemia, 72
Idioventricular rhythm, 40
In-custody death syndrome, 20, 34
Institute of Non-Lethal Defense
Technologies, 45
International Association of
Chiefs of Police, 3, 148, 194
International Classification of
Diseases, 16
International Statistical
Classification of Diseases
and Related Health Issues,
10th Revision, 33
Joint Non-Lethal Weapons Human
Effects Center of Excellence,
50
Ketamine, 29
Ketoacidosis, 25
Kraeplin, Emil, 33
Lactate, 73, 76-85
Lethal force, 5, 8, 149
Levacetylmethadol, 30
Lysergic acid diethylamide, 10,
30-31, 95-96, 117-118, 131,
135, 140, 143

Marijuana, 9-10, 29, 67, 95-96, 115, 117, 119, 131, 135, 140, 143

Mental illness, 11-13, 17, 20, 31-34, 100-103, 108, 116, 122, 125-128, 131, 135-136, 143, 145, 147-148, 150, 153-155, 158

Mentally ill, *See* Mental illness

Meperidine, 30

Methadone, 30

Methamphetamine, 24, 27-28, 34, 48-49, 95

Minister of Health, 34

Minister of Justice, 34

Minute ventilation, 72, 74, 78

Mitral valve prolapse, 78

Monomorphic premature ventricular complexes, 60

Myocardial infarction, 27-29, 66, 71, 78

Myocardial ischemia, 75

Myocardial necrosis, 53, 62

Myocardium, 44, 71

Myoglobin, 77-78

Naranjo algorithm, 5

National Association of Medical Examiners, 34

National Survey on Drug Use and Health, 31

National Violent Death Reporting System, 19

Nervous system
Autonomic, 26
Central, 3, 28
Peripheral, 3
Somatic, 3
Sympathetic, 26

Ninth Judicial District Court of Appeals, 6

Norepinephrine, 35, 84

Office of the Chief Coroner for Ontario, 11

Oleoresin capsicum, 82-85

Opiate, 10, 30, 117, 119-120, 131, 135, 140, 143

Opium, 30

Oxycodone, 30

Oxymorphone, 30

Pacemaker, 11-13, 17, 19, 67-71, 87, 95, 97, 100, 102-103, 108, 115, 128, 131, 134, 140, 148, 156

Partial pressure of carbon dioxide, 72-73, 76-82

Partial pressure of oxygen, 72-73, 77-81

Peak loaded voltage, 2

Pectoralis major, 40

Phencyclidine, 10, 29-30, 95-96, 117, 120, 131, 135, 140, 143

Phrenic nerve, 72-73

Police Executive Research Forum, 5, 13, 149

Positional asphyxia, 35

Potassium, 73, 75, 77, 79-80, 85

Premature ventricular contraction, 40, 56

Prime implicants, 130-131, 136

Product liability, 153

Pseudo-monophasic waveform, 2-3, 51, 77

Psychotropic medications, 14, 17, 19, 85, 87, 97, 100, 102-103, 108, 116, 126-128, 136, 140, 147, 156, 158

Pulseless electrical activity, 40, 64, 65
Purkinje fibers, 41
QRS complex, 32
QT prolongation, 32
Qualitative Comparative Analysis, 88, 101, 127, 157
Radiofrequency ablation, 41
Respiratory rate, 72-74, 77-78
R-wave, 43
Schizophrenia, 29, 31, 35, 71, 96
Sertürner, Frederich, 30
Shulak, N. R., 34
Sinus rhythm, 45, 57-58, 60-61, 63-64, 66, 68, 95
Sinus tachycardia, 49, 56-58, 66, 70
Sodium, 27, 73, 75, 77
Strength-duration formula, 49
Stroke, 27
Sudden death, 2, 8, 10, 16-17, 20-22, 25-26, 29, 31-32, 35, 78, 81-82, 85, 87-89, 91-92, 98, 100, 102-103, 110, 112-114, 116-124, 126-127, 133-134, 139, 145, 148-149, 156-157
Supreme Court, 93, 151
Sympathetic-adrenal-medulla axis, 75, 82-83
Sympathomimetic, 26, 28, 35, 81
Tachyarrhythmia, 60, 62

Tachycardia, 61, 69, 76
TASER International, Inc., 1, 3, 6, 39-40, 153-154
Task Force on Electronic Weapons, 8, 12
The Pennsylvania State University, 45
Tidal volume, 72-74, 78
Torsade de pointes, 32
Tramadol, 30
Troponin I, 44, 59, 62-63, 66, 82
T-wave, 32, 43, 48, 52
Ultrasonography, 60-61, 63, 73
Ultrasound, 60
Uniform Crime Reports, 4, 23
United Nations, 16
Ventricular fibrillation, 9, 22, 28, 32, 39-55, 64-65, 67-70, 76
Ventricular tachycardia, 9, 25, 44-45, 49, 55, 64, 67, 70-71
Weapons
   Less-lethal, 5, 16-17, 149-150
   Non-lethal, 5
Wide-Ranging Online Data for Epidemiologic Research, 19
World Health Organization, 16
Wrongful death, 5, 14, 91, 150, 154
Xiphoid process, 77

CPSIA information can be obtained at www.ICGtesting.com
Printed in the USA
BVOW02*1804030215

385257BV00002B/3/P

DATE DUE	RETURNED
NOV 2 2 2010	